O U L

OXFORD UROLOGY LIBRARY

Benign Prostatic Hyperplasia and Lower Urinary Tract Symptoms in Men

D1423678

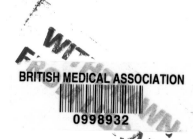

▶ Except where otherwise stated, drug doses and recommendations are for the non-pregnant adult who is not breast-feeding.

O U L

OXFORD UROLOGY LIBRARY

Benign Prostatic Hyperplasia and Lower Urinary Tract Symptoms in Men

Edited by

Alexander Bachmann

Head of Department of Urology
University Hospital Basel
University of Basel
Switzerland

Jean J.M.C.H. de la Rosette

Professor of Urology and
Head Department of Urology
AMC University Hospital
Amsterdam, The Netherlands

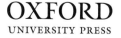

OXFORD
UNIVERSITY PRESS

OXFORD
UNIVERSITY PRESS

Great Clarendon Street, Oxford OX2 6DP

Oxford University Press is a department of the University of Oxford.
It furthers the University's objective of excellence in research, scholarship,
and education by publishing worldwide in

Oxford New York

Auckland Cape Town Dar es Salaam Hong Kong Karachi
Kuala Lumpur Madrid Melbourne Mexico City Nairobi
New Delhi Shanghai Taipei Toronto

With offices in

Argentina Austria Brazil Chile Czech Republic France Greece
Guatemala Hungary Italy Japan Poland Portugal Singapore
South Korea Switzerland Thailand Turkey Ukraine Vietnam

Oxford is a registered trade mark of Oxford University Press
in the UK and in certain other countries

Published in the United States
by Oxford University Press Inc., New York

© Oxford University Press 2012

British Library Cataloguing in Publication Data

Data available

Library of Congress Cataloging in Publication Data

Data available

Typeset by Cenveo, Bangalore, India
Printed in Great Britain
on acid-free paper by
Ashford Colour Press Ltd, Gosport, Hampshire

ISBN 978–0–19–957277–9

10 9 8 7 6 5 4 3 2 1

Whilst every effort has been made to ensure that the contents of this book
are as complete, accurate and-up-to-date as possible at the date of writing.
Oxford University Press is not able to give any guarantee or assurance that
such is the case. Readers are urged to take appropriately qualified medical
advice in all cases. The information in this book is intended to be useful to the
general reader, but should not be used as a means o self-diagnosis or for the
prescription of medication.

Contents

Foreword *ix*
Preface *xi*
Symbols and abbreviations *xiii*
Contributors *xvii*

1. Definitions: LUTS, BPH, BPE, BOO, BPO | 1
2. Natural history of untreated BPH and its impact on LUTS | 7
3. Pathophysiology of BPH, symptoms, and symptom scores | 17
4. BPH, PSA, and the risk of having prostate cancer (PCA) | 25
5. Erectile dysfunction associated with LUTS and BPH | 33
6. OAB, LUTS, and BPH—a paradigm shift | 37
7. Bladder outflow obstruction, urodynamic studies and BPH | 43
8. Aging men and LUTS | 49
9. Risk factors associated with BPH | 53
10. Diagnosis and assessment of BPH: subjective parameters | 59
11. Diagnosis and assessment of BPH: objective parameters | 65

12. Watchful waiting and lifestyle issues
    associated with LUTS and BPH 79

13. Medical treatment of LUTS and BPH 85

14. Interventional treatment: open prostatectomy 95

15. Interventional treatment: transurethral
    resection of the prostate (TURP) 101

16. Interventional treatment: Prostate laser 109

17. Interventional treatment: Greenlight laser 115

18. Interventional treatment: Holmium laser 121

19. Interventional treatment: Thulium laser 127

20. Interventional treatment: Diode laser 131

21. Risk-adapted management of BPH 137

22. Complications of BPH 147

23. Algorithms in the management of benign
    prostatic hyperplasia   163

24. Emergencies due to BPH   169

    Index 177

Foreword

Benign prostatic hyperplasia (BPH) causing lower urinary tract symptoms (LUTS) in men continues to occupy time of most urologists. There has been a considerable advancement in our knowledge of the condition, both the natural history, the cause of the symptoms, the appropriate investigations, the medical management and the minimally invasive treatment of the condition. We are now in a better position to know which patient will respond better to appropriate medical management and what the likely outcome might be. Transurethral resection of the prostate has been the standard method of treating obstructive BPH for many years and there have been a number of recent modifications of this relating to the introduction of different diathermy technology. Whether these changes will have a large and lasting impact on the treatment of this condition remains to be seen. There has been a huge number of interventional treatments for obstructive BPH, many of which have been disgarded, but the use of the laser continues to be of interest and produced many interesting papers which have been published in the world of literature. The Editors of this book are to be congratulated on assembling an outstanding group of authors, all well recognised names who are leaders in this field. The book itself should be on considerable interest with each section being briefly and succinctly written, for ready and immediate access for the reader. I feel that the book will help clinicians in their treatment of BPH and LUTS in men and feel that it is of potential importance for trainees as well as Urologists who look after patients with this condition.

John M. Fitzpatrick MCh FRCSI FC Urol (SA) FRCSGlas FRCS
Consultant Urologist and Professor of Surgery

Preface

Diagnosis and treatment of so called benign prostatic hyperplasia (BPH) is considered to be one of the most important topics in urology and afflicts millions of aged men world-wide, as there is a significant relationship between having lower urinary tract symptoms (LUTS) due to progressive prostatic growth, histological benign prostatic enlargement and age, potentially each men could be afflicted with. Although it is not life threatening, it is a clinical manifestation that reduces a patient's quality of life over many years. Beside the high economical burden impacting potentially each aging man, patients often suffering from LUTS due to BPH and associated complaints for a very long time.

This book will cover several topics including definitions and coherences, incidence and prevalence of BPH, over-active bladder (OAB) and issues of erectile dysfunction. Additionally, risk factors, diagnostic- and assessment tools, PSA topics, watchful-waiting issues, lifestyle aspects, medical and surgical treatment options are covered. As in the last few years plenty of new minimally-invasive surgical treatment options are emerging on the market, a comprehensive and structured overview is given. Furthermore treatment recommendations, especially for patients under special conditions including cardio-pulmonal co-morbidities are given. Finally a risk adapted management, general treatment algorithm and complications associated with BPH are discussed.

This book of BPH and LUTS in men is addressed to general practitioners, students, urological interested physicians and physician who wish to increase their urological horizon beyond their own specialized expertise. Beside a short and concise clinical and pathophysiological background the newest update of general and specialized treatment options, including evaluation of the most emerging surgical techniques is given.

It was a really pleasure for us to have invited many key opinion leaders on their dedicated field.

Basel, January 2011
Alexander Bachmann

Amsterdam, January 2011
Jean J.M.C.H. de la Rosette

Symbols and abbreviations

5ARI	5α-reductase inhibitor
AAH	atypical adenomatous hyperplasia
AB	alphablockers
AG	Abrams-Griffiths
ANS	autonomic nervous system
ARB	α_1-adrenoceptor receptor antagonist
AUA	American Urological Association
AUA-SI	American Urological Association Symptom Index
AUR	acute urinary retention
BACH	Boston Area Community Health
CLAP	contact laser ablation of the prostate
DM	diabetes mellitus type II
BOO	bladder outlet obstruction
BPE	benign prostatic enlargement
BPH	benign prostatic hyperplasia
BPO	benign prostatic obstruction
CNS	central nervous system
CombAT	combination of Avodart and Tamsulosin study
CPPS	chronic pelvic pain syndrome
DAN-PSS	Danish Prostatic Symptom Score
DO	detrusor overactivity
DRE	digital rectal examination
DUA	detrusor underactivity
ED	erectile dysfunction
EMG	electromyography
EPIC	European Prospective Investigation into Cancer and Nutrition
ER	estrogen receptors
HoLEP	Holmium laser enucleation

HoLRP	Holmium:YAG laser
ICIQ-MLUTS	International Consultation on Incontinence Modular Questionnaire-male Lower Urinary Tract Symptoms
ICS	International Continence Society
ILC	interstitial laser coagulation
IPSS	international prostate symptom score
KTP	potassium-titanyl-phosphate
LBO	Lithium triborat
LinPURR	linear passive urethral resistance relation
LUTS	lower urinary tract symptoms
MRI	magnetic resonance imaging
MSA	multiple system atrophy
MTOPS	medical therapy of prostatic symptoms
Nd:YAG	Neodymium:Yttrium-Aluminium-Garnet
NOS	nitric oxide synthase
OAB	overactive bladder
OP	open prostatectomy
PCA	prostate cancer
PD	Parkinson's disease
PDE-5	phosphodiesterase
PFS	pressure/flow studies
PIA	proliferative inflammatory atrophy
PSA	prostate specific antigen
PV	prostatic volume
PVDT	prostate volume doubling time
PVP	photoselective vaporization of the prostate
PVR	postvoidal residual urine
QoL	quality of life
RCT	randomized controlled trials
TRUS	transrectal ultrasound
TUIP	transurethral incision of the prostate
TUMT	transurethral microwave therapy
TUNA	transurethral needle ablation (of the prostate)
TURP	transurethral resection of the prostate
TWOC	trial without catheter

TZ	transition zone
UTI	urinary tract infection
VLAP	visually assisted laser prostatectomy
WW	watchful waiting

Contributors

Karl-Erik Andersson

Professor of Urology and
Clinical Pharmacology
Institute for Regenerative
Medicine
Wake Forest University School
of Medicine
Medical Center Boulevard
Winston-Salem, United States

Alexander Bachmann

Professor of Urology and
Chairman
Department of Urology
University Hospital Basel,
University of Basel
Basel, Switzerland

Ingrid Becker

Fellow of Urology
Department of Urology and
Andrology Donauspital
Vienna, Austria

Reginald Bruskewitz

Professor Emeritus
Department of Urology
University of Wisconsin
UW Medical Foundation
Madison, United States

Professor Lukas Bubendorf

Professor of Pathology
Institute for Pathology,
University of Basel
Basel, Switzerland

Stephan Degener

Associate Professor of Urology
Department of Urology
University Medical Center
Witten/Herdecke, Germany

Judith Dockray

Clinical Research Fellow
Department of Urology
King's College Hospital
London, UK

**Professor Thomas C.
Gasser**

Professor of Urology and
Chairman
Department of Urology
University Hospital Basel,
Basel, Switzerland

Peter J. Gilling

Professor of Urology and
Chairman, F.R.A.C.S.
Department of Urology
Promed Urology
Tauranga, New Zealand

Dr C. Gratzke

Associate Professor of Urology
Department of Urology
University Hospital,
Ludwig Maximilians University,
Munich, Germany

Stavros Gravas

Assistant Professor
Department of Urology
University of Thessaly
Larissa, Greece

Professor Andreas J. Gross

Professor of Urology
Department of Urology
Asklepios Klinik Barmbek
Hamburg, Germany

Seife Hailemariam
Institut of Histological and
Cytological Diagnostics
Aarau, Switzerland

Julia Heinzelbecker
Resident
Department of Urology
University Medical Center
Mannheim, Germany

Thomas Hermanns
Resident
Divison of Urology
University of Zürich
University Hospital
Zürich, Switzerland

Professor Herbert Leyh
Professor of Urology and
Director
Department of Urology
Klinikum Garmisch-
Partenkirchen
Garmisch-Partenkirchen,
Germany

Stephan Madersbacher
Associate Professor of Urology
Department of Urology and
Andrology Donauspital
Vienna, Austria

Michael J. Mathers
Urological Ambulatory
Remscheid
in cooperation with the
Department of Urology
HELIOS Klinikum Wuppertal
University Medical Center
Witten/Herdecke, Germany

Professor Martin C. Michel
Professor of Pharmacology
and Director Department
of Pharmacology &
Pharmacotherapy Academic
Medical Center
Amsterdam, The Netherlands

**Professor Maurice
Stephan Michel**
Professor of Urology and
Chairman
Department of Urology,
University Medical Center
Mannheim, Germany

Mr Gordon H. Muir
Consultant Urological Surgeon,
King's College Hospital
Honorary Senior Lecturer,
King's College, UK

Jørgen Nordling
Clinical Professor
Department of Urology
Herlev Hospital,
University of Copenhagen
Herlev, Denmark

Matthias Oelke
Associate Professor of Urology
Department of Urology
Hannover Medical School
Hannover, Germany

Professor Jens J. Rassweiler
Professor of Urology, Dr. h. c.
and Director
Department of Urology
SLK-Kliniken Heilbronn GmbH
Heilbronn, Germany

Dr Oliver Reich
Associate Professor of Urology
and Director
Department of Urology
Klinikum Harlaching
Munich, Germany

Malte Riethen
Resident
Department of Urology
University Hospital Basel
University of Basel
Basel, Switzerland

Alexander Roosen
Resident
Department of Urology
University Hospital Munich
Ludwig Maximilians University
Munich, Germany

Jean J.M.C.H. de la Rosette
Professor of Urology and Head
Department of Urology
AMC University Hospital
Amsterdam, The Netherlands

Dr Michael Seitz
Associate Professor of Urology
and Vice-Chairman
Department of Urology
University Hospital
Ludwig-Maximilians-University
Munich, Germany

Frank Sommer
Professor of Urology
Institute for Men's Health
University Hospital
Hamburg, Germany

Professor Christian G. Stief
Professor of Urology and
Chairman
Department of Urology
University Hospital Munich,
Campus GrosshadernLudwig
Maximilians-University Munich,
Munich, Germany

Professor Tullio Sulser
Professor of Urology and
Chairman
Divison of UrologyUniversity
of Zurich
Zürich, Switzerland

Derya Tilki
Associate Professor of Urology
Department of Urology
University Hospital,
Ludwig Maximilians University,
Munich, Germany

Liam C. Wilson
Consultant Urologist
Department of Urology
Tauranga Hospital
Tauranga, New Zealand

Dr Stephen F. Wyler
Associate Professor of Urology
Department of Urology
University Hospital Basel,
University of Basel
Basel, Switzerland

Chapter 1

Definitions: LUTS, BPH, BPE, BOO, BPO

Jean de la Rosette

> **Key points**
> - LUTS are the subjective indicator of a disease
> - LUTS can be classified as storage, voiding and post micturition symptoms
> - LUTS cannot be used for defined diagnosis
> - The coherence of LUTS (symptoms), BPO (urodynamic), BPE (pathological) and BPM (histological) is not fully understood.

Historically, a number of terms such as prostatism, symptomatic benign prostatic hyperplasia (BPH), and clinical BPH have been used to describe symptoms related to micturition in older men. Nowadays, the traditional belief that urinary symptoms in elderly men were always assumed to be directly or indirectly related to prostate has been challenged. The term lower urinary tract symptoms (LUTS) has been adopted and several consensus and guidelines committees have attempted to define the appropriate terminology for categorizing the pathophysiological conditions underlying male LUTS.

   LUTS (as defined by the International Continence Society) are the subjective indicator of a disease or change in condition as perceived by the patient, caregiver or partner and may lead him/her to seek help from health care professionals. LUTS can be classified as storage, voiding, and post micturition symptoms.

- ***Bladder storage (irritative) symptoms*** are experienced during the storage phase of the bladder and include: increased daytime frequency, nocturia, urgency, and urinary incontinence

- **Voiding (obstructive) urinary symptoms** are experienced during the voiding phase and include: slow urinary stream, splitting or spraying of the urinary stream, intermittent urinary stream, hesitancy, straining to void, and terminal dribbling
- **Post micturition symptoms** include feeling of incomplete emptying and postmicturition dribbling.

> LUTS cannot be used to make a definitive diagnosis.

- **Benign prostatic hyperplasia (BPH)** represents a histologic diagnosis that refers to the proliferation of smooth muscle and epithelial cells within the prostatic transition zone. Therefore, BPH is a term used (and reserved for) the typical histological pattern which defines the disease
- **Benign prostatic enlargement (BPE)** is defined as prostatic enlargement due to histologic benign prostatic hyperplasia. The term "prostatic enlargement" should be used in the absence of prostatic histology
- **Bladder outlet obstruction (BOO)** is the generic term for obstruction during voiding and is characterized by increased detrusor pressure and reduced urine flow rate. Therefore, the term BOO requires urodynamic confirmation
- **Benign prostatic obstruction (BPO)** is a form of bladder outlet obstruction (needs urodynamic evaluation) and may be diagnosed when the cause of outlet obstruction is known to be benign prostatic enlargement, due to histologic benign prostatic hyperplasia.

> It should be underlined that the use of incorrect and inconsistent terminology may lead to confusion among clinicians and patients and mismanagement of the conditions that underlie male LUTS.

1.1 Epidemiology

Despite the high impact of BPH on public health, a standard and globally accepted epidemiological definition of BPH remains controversial, making the study of epidemiology and natural history of the disease difficult. Prevalence and incidence rates must be viewed in the context of the definition criteria chosen by the different authors.

- Prevalence has been calculated on the basis of histological criteria (autopsy prevalence) or clinical criteria (clinical prevalence). The age-specific autopsy prevalence has been shown to be relatively consistent around the world, regardless ethnicity. A histological prevalence of 10% at the age of 30, 20% at the age of 40, 50%–60% at the age of 60, and 80%–90% at the age of 70 and 80 was reported.

However, many men with histological BPH will never seek for help, nor do they need any treatment for it. The condition becomes a clinical entity when it is associated with LUTS. Most of the clinic-based studies on BPH epidemiology have been conducted in cohorts of symptomatic men presenting to urologists or primary care physicians. These studies may be biased due to recruitment criteria.

In addition, the historical epidemiological studies lack of a uniform definition of clinical BPH, quantitative instruments for assessing LUTS severity, a noninvasive, and accurate method for measuring prostate volume and bladder outlet obstruction make the interpretation of the data more difficult.

Another limitation was the lack of consensus regarding prostate size or obstructed bladder. Later on, the development of instruments measuring the severity of LUTS, prostate volume, and urodynamic parameters, provided the opportunity to define prevalence rates in the general male community accurately.

Thus, many investigators designed cross sectional studies to determine the prevalence of clinical BPH. Patients were diagnosed as having clinical BPH if the IPSS score was ≥8, peak flow rate was <15 mL/sec, and prostate volume 20 cm³. This definition of clinical BPH shows the prevalence of the disease to be consistently age-related.

> In the Olmstead County survey one of the largest and longest running longitudinal study showed that moderate-to-severe symptoms can occur among 13% of men aged 40–49 years and among 28% of those older than 70 years.

1.2 **Progression**

BPH progression is a dynamic process that includes deterioration of LUTS and health related quality of life, increased prostatic size, acute urinary retention (AUR), and BPH-related surgery. Renal insufficiency and recurrent urinary tract infections as additional measures of BPH progression have also been considered. However, these outcomes are rarely observed.

> Data from longitudinal population-based studies best analyze the natural history of diseases because of limited selection criteria and the data from placebo arms of controlled studies, However, the bias from the strict inclusion criteria provides strong evidence that BPH is a progressive disease.

- In the Olmsted County Study, an average increase in the IPSS of 0.18 points/year, a decrease in peak flow rate of 2%/year and a median prostate growth of 1.9%/year was observed in a randomly selected cohort of 2,115 men aged 40–79 years followed for 12 years
- In the placebo arm of the Medical Therapy of Prostatic Symptoms (MTOPS) study the rate of overall clinical progression was 17.4% over the 4-year duration of the study. About 78% of progression events were referred as deterioration in symptoms.

1.3 Coherences

The relationship between LUTS, BPH, BPE, BOO and BPO is complex and not fully understood. Because the prevalence of histological BPH and LUTS is age-related, it was often assumed that they were causally related, but recent evidence indicate that male LUTS may result from a complex interplay of pathophysiological influences, including prostatic pathology and bladder dysfunction. However, BPH is the primary cause of LUTS in older men.

BPE occurs in some but not all men with BPH and LUTS, and some men with enlarged prostates may not have any symptoms at all. Of men with BPE, some but again not all develop BOO which is characterized by increased detrusor pressure and reduced urine flow rate.

BOO due to BPE have both static (increased tissue mass) and dynamic (increased smooth muscle tone) components in the prostate. BPE can also lead to overactivity of the detrusor muscle.

> Physicians should use the term LUTS to describe symptoms and use the terms BPH, BPE, and BOO once diagnosis is confirmed by appropriate diagnostic procedures, e.g. "LUTS due to BPH, or BPE or BOOs".

References

Abrams P, Cardozo L, Fall M, Griffiths D, Rosier P, Ulmsten U, Van Kerrebroeck P, Victor A, Wein A (2003) Standardisation Sub-Committee of the International Continence Society. The standardisation of terminology in lower urinary tract function: report from the standardisation sub-committee of the International Continence Society *Urology* **61**: 37–49.

Arrighi HM, Metter EJ, Guess HA, Fozzard JL (1991) Natural history of benign prostatic hyperplasia and risk of prostatectomy, the Baltimore Longitudinal Study of Aging *Urology* **35**(Suppl): 4–8.

Chapple CR, Roehrborn CG (2006) A shifted paradigm for the further understanding, evaluation, and treatment of lower urinary tract symptoms in men: focus on the bladder *Eur Urol* **49**: 651–8.

Chute CG, Panser LA, Girman CJ, Oesterling JE, Guess HA, Jacobsen SJ, Lieber MM (1993) The prevalence of prostatism: a population based survey of urinary symptoms *J Urol* **150**: 85–9.

Emberton M, Andriole GL, de la Rosette J et al. (2003) Benign prostatic hyperplasia: a progressive disease of aging men *Urology* **61**: 267–73.

Issa MM, Fenter TC, Black L, Grogg AL, Kruep EJ (2006) An assessment of the diagnosed prevalence of diseases in men 50 years of age or older. *Am J Manag Care* **12**: S83–9.

Jacobsen SJ, Girman CJ, Guess HA et al. (1996) Natural history of prostatism: longitudinal changes in voiding symptoms in community dwelling men *J Urol* **155**: 595–600.

McConnell JD, Roehrborn CG, Bautista OM et al. (2003) The long-term effect of doxazosin, finasteride, and combination therapy on the clinical progression of benign prostatic hyperplasia *N Engl J Med* **349**: 2387–98.

Roberts RO, Jacobsen SJ, Jacobsen D et al. (2000) Longitudinal changes in peak urinary flow rates in a community based cohort *J Urol* **163**: 107–13.

Roehrborn CG (2005) Benign prostatic hyperplasia: An overview *Rev Urol* **7**(9): S3–14.

Chapter 2

Natural history of untreated BPH and its impact on LUTS

Karl-Erik Andersson

> **Key points**
>
> - Histologic BPH is a progressive disease, dependent on age and androgen
> - The morbidity of histologic BPH is manifested by LUTS and/or outcome events (e.g. AUR)
> - LUTS are age-related, but progression over time in individuals is highly variable
> - Although both histologic BPH and LUTS are are age-dependent and progressive, this does not necessarily mean that they share the same pathophysiology or a common time course.

Benign prostatic hyperplasia (BPH) is a histological diagnosis, based on microscopic evidence of prostatic stromal and epithelial hyperplasia (Table 2.1). However, the triad of prostatic hyperplasia with benign enlargement of the gland (BPE), benign prostatic obstruction (BPO), and lower urinary tract symptoms (LUTS), is the basis for the clinical diagnosis of BPH (Figure 2.1).

LUTS include storage, voiding, and post-micturition symptoms (Abrams et al., 2002), and occur commonly in both men and women, and can therefore not be specifically prostate related. What is then the contribution of changes in the prostate to LUTS and how does the natural history of histologic BPH impact on the pathogenesis and development of LUTS?

Fig 2.1 Consequences of histological BPH and components of the clinical diagnosis

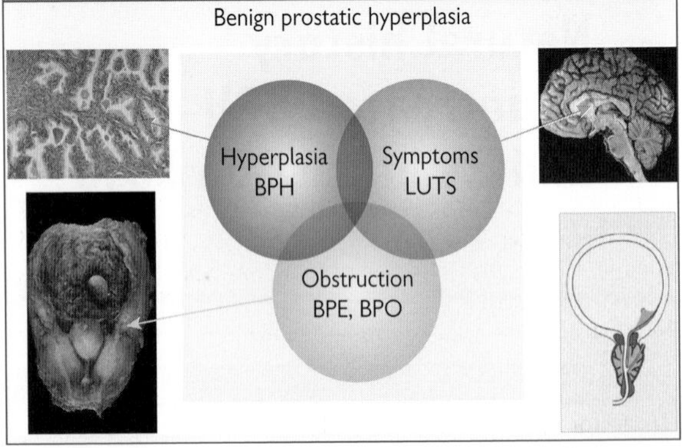

Benign prostatic hyperplasia

Hyperplasia BPH

Symptoms LUTS

Obstruction BPE, BPO

Table 2.1 Terminology

- BPH = benign prostatic hyperplasia. Histological diagnosis requiring examination of prostate samples obtained at autopsy, biopsy, or surgery
- BPE = benign prostatic enlargement. Can be assessed by digital rectal examination (DRE), transrectal ultrasound (TRUS), magnetic resonance imaging (MRI), prostate specific antigen (PSA)
- BPO = benign prostatic obstruction. Can be assessed by pressure-flow studies and flow rates
- LUTS = lower urinary tract symptoms.

2.1 Natural history and epidemiology of (untreated) BPH

The natural history of a disease refers to the progression of the untreated disease over time. The natural history of BPH is incompletely understood because of the absence of a uniform definition of the disease and the lack of rigorous studies. The prevalence of histologic BPH can be determined from autopsy studies, biopsies, or surgery (Table 2.2) and seems to be similar throughout the world.

- More than two-thirds of men older than 50 years were found to have histological evidence of BPH and, after age 70 years, the proportion increased to more than 80%. The logistic growth curve of BPH lesions removed at prostatectomy indicated that the growth of BPH is initiated probably before the age of 30 years (Berry et al., 1984).

Table 2.2 Morbidity of histological BPH
• LUTS = lower urinary tract symptoms
• AUR = acute urinary retention
• UTI = urinary tract infection
Obstructive kidney disease (rare).

A surrogate means for identifying and study the development of BPH and prostate growth is assessment of prostatic volume (PV). Confirming the results of several previous reports, Lieber et al. (2009) found in a large sample of community living men that the annual increase of PV was 2.2%. Lieber et al. (2009), found PV doubling time (PVDT) a useful measure of prostate growth.

> The factor most strongly associated with prostate volume doubling time is baseline transition zone volume.

It is generally considered that PV overall increases with age, however, Lieber et al. (2009) found that PVDT, reflecting the rate of prostate growth, was not age-dependent.

- The morbidity of histological BPH is manifested by LUTS and/or outcome events, such as acute urinary retention, urinary tract infection, and rarely, obstructive kidney disease (Table 2.2). The clinical consequences have been assessed by a number of investigators in epidemiological and clinical studies using various scales, e.g. the American Urological Association Symptom Index (AUASI) and the International Prostate Symptom Score (IPSS), and urinary flow rates.
- One of the best known studies is the Olmsted County Study that was initiated in 1990 (see, e.g. Fitzpatrick, 2006). For 12 years a randomly selected cohort of 2,115 men aged 40–79 years was followed. At inclusion, 26% of men aged 40–49 years had moderate to severe LUTS, and this increased to 46% in men aged 70–79 years. There was a mean increase in the IPSS of 0.18 points per year, ranging from 0.05 in men in their forties to 0.44 in men in their sixties. The median peak flow rate decreased from 21.2 mL/s to 14.2 mL/s in men in the respective age groups. At the follow-up, the severity of LUTS increased and the peak flow rate decreased with time and age. The decrease in median peak flow rate of 2.1% per year was also age-related, with men aged ≥70 years showing a more rapid decline (6.2% per year) than men in their fifties (1.1% per year).

Table 2.3 Pathophysiology of LUTS

- Androgen/estrogen signaling imbalance
- Aging
- Embryonic re-awakening
- Stem cell defects
- Chronic inflammation
- Increase TGF-b signalling
- Adrenergic hyperactivity
- Undefined factors.

2.2 Pathophysiology of (untreated) BPH

The specific factors that initiate and promote the proliferative process of histologic BPH are unknown but requires androgens and aging (Table 2.3). Males with 5a-reductase deficiency and males who are castrated early in life do not develop BPH, except of very rare reports (Brown J.A. et al., 1997, Casella et al., 2005).

In patients without testosteron deprivation levels a possible explanation for the development of BPH could be mutations of the androgen receptor; this in analogy to the progression of prostate cancer after androgen withdrawal. Due to these mutations, the androgen receptor can 'normally' work even in nearby complete absence of androgens (Casella, 2005).

McNeal (1978) postulated that BPH results from an awakening of embryonic inductive interactions between the prostatic stroma and the epithelium, which in turn induces epithelial hyperplasia. He proposed that the initial lesion of BPH is not a stromal nodule but a formation of glandular budding and branching toward a central focus that occurs primarily in the transition zone, a situation reminiscent of embryonic development. Whether abnormal growth in BPH is due to embryonic reawakening, stem cell defects, chronic inflammation, imbalance between androgen/estrogen signalling, increased TGF-b signalling, adrenergic overactivity, or to other so-far undefined factors, is an area of intense investigation.

2.3 Natural history and epidemiology of (untreated) LUTS

The prevalence of LUTS is known to be age-related, however, the natural history of LUTS in is poorly understood (Table 2.3). Lee et al. (1998) assessed the natural history of LUTS in 1994 men, aged 40–79 years, followed up for a period of 5 years. Although the progression of LUTS over time in individual men was very variable, the overall trend was one of continuing deterioration. Temml et al. (2003) assessed the natural history of LUTS in a cohort of 456 previously untreated men, aged 40–84 years, followed for 5 years. There was a slow progression and mean IPSS increase from 4.6 to 5.5 years, but not all LUTS progressed in a similar way.

> Thus, storage symptoms had a higher tendency to improve over time.

- Several recent studies have established that the prevalence of LUTS increases with age in both men and women (Irwin et al., 2006; Kupelian et al., 2006; Coyne et al., 2009). Estimating the prevalence of urinary incontinence (UI), overactive bladder (OAB), and other LUTS among 19,165 men and women in five countries using the 2002 International Continence Society (ICS) definitions, Irwin et al. found that 64.3% reported at least one LUTS. Nocturia was the most prevalent LUTS (men, 48.6%; women, 54.5%). The prevalence of storage LUTS (men, 51.3%; women, 59.2%) was greater than that for voiding (men, 25.7%; women, 19.5%) and postmicturition (men, 16.9%; women, 14.2%) symptoms combined.

- Kupelian et al. (2009) presented a population-based epidemiological survey of a broad range of urological symptoms and risk factors among randomly selected 5,503 adults aged 30–79 years in three race/ethnic groups (Black, Hispanian, White), recruited in the city of Boston (the BACH study). The controls provided for effects of gender, race/ ethnicity, and socio-economic status. The overall prevalence of LUTS (AUA Symptom Index, SI, of ≥8) was 18.7% and increased with age (10.5% for 30–39 years to 25.5% for 70–79 years), but did not differ by gender or race/ ethnicity. Voiding symptoms occurred more frequently in men, but the prevalence of storage symptoms was generally higher than voiding symptoms for both men and women.

> Voiding symptoms occurred more frequently in men, but the prevalence of storage symptoms was generally higher than voiding symptoms for both men and women.

- The EpiLUTS study was a cross-sectional, population representative, Internet-based survey conducted in the USA, the UK and Sweden in 30,000 men and women aged 40–99 years (mean 56.6) to assess the prevalence and associated bother of LUTS (Coyne et al., 2009). When LUTS were reported often or more frequently, 47.9% of male and 52.5% of female respondents reported at least one LUTS. Although voiding symptoms occurred more frequently in men, the prevalence of storage symptoms was generally higher than voiding symptoms for both men and women.

> The prevalence of all LUTS increased with age in men, but only urgency, urgency with fear of leaking, weak stream, urgency incontinence, and nocturnal enuresis increased with age in women.

2.4 Pathophysiology of LUTS

Voiding (obstructive) LUTS have been attributed to two factors:
- the physical mass of the enlarged gland (the static component) and
- the tone of the smooth muscle of the prostatic stroma (the dynamic component). Storage (irritative) LUTS, on the other hand, have been associated with bladder dysfunction produced by BPO. It is reasonable to expect a relation between voiding LUTS and prostate size. Indeed, population-based studies have demonstrated modest correlations between BPE, BPO (Jacobsen et al., 2001), and LUTS, but evidence for a direct link between these entities is far from convincing.

It is now recognized that LUTS do not reliably reflect the underlying vesico-urethral pathology, and that other factors than BPE and BPO can cause LUTS (Andersson, 2003)

> Increasing experimental evidence suggests that the bladder has to be considered the central organ in the pathogenesis of storage LUTS, not only in women, but also in men (Table 2.4).

A relation between voiding LUTS and BPO seems reasonable, but BPO cannot be the only contributor.
- Storage symptoms have a close association with underlying detrusor overactivity (DO). Several theories on the mechanisms of DO have been put forward and have focused on the urothelium and on myogenic and neurogenic factors (Andersson, 2009; Rosen et al., 2009). However, each of these factors probably contributes in varying proportion to the genesis of DO and the associated storage LUTS, including overactive bladder (OAB).

Table 2.4 Factors affecting bladder function and LUTS

- Local factors
- Hormonal changes
- Bladder outlet obstruction
- Aging
- Ischemia
- High nocturnal diuresis
- Concomitant diseases
- Neurologic diseases.

2.5 Impact of natural history of BPH on LUTS

Several studies have attempted to estimate the prevalence of the clinical consequences of histologic BPH by determining the presence of LUTS suggestive of BPO associated with BPH. Wei et al. (2005) estimated that 6.5 million of 27 million white men aged 50–79 years in the USA met the criteria for discussion of potential treatment for BPH in the year 2000 (Wei et al., 2005).

- In outpatients aged ≥40 years who were users of Department of Veteran Affairs health care services, the prevalence of BPH/LUTS was 4.8% (Anger et al., 2008). Using the criteria of an IPSS of >7, 42% of men aged ≥50 years and visiting their primary-care physician for routine care had LUTS suggestive of BPH (Naslund et al., 2006). Figures ranging from 16.1 to 57.5% have been reported from other countries (Kaplan et al., 2009).

- The clinically important parameters of disease progression in men with moderate to severe LUTS and low peak flow rates are symptom progression and the development of acute urinary retention (AUR). The risk of AUR is related to both baseline serum PSA level and prostate volume.

Both histologic BPH and LUTS are progressive conditions that are age dependent. This does not necessarily mean that the two conditions share the same pathophysiology or a common time course.

- The pathophysiology, epidemiology, and natural history of both BPH and LUTS are incompletely understood. The impact of histological BPH on LUTS has not been established, but prostate growth rate, as reflected by prostate volume doubling time, makes it reasonable to assume that patients with rapid prostate growth are more likely to develop bothersome LUTS. It is important to recognize that many other factors unrelated to BPE and BPO are involved in the pathophysiology of LUTS. Although LUTS, BPE, and BPO are age-dependent, they are not necessarily causally related. At the individual level, the natural histories of these parameters are highly variable.

References

Abrams P, Cardozo L, Fall M, Griffiths D, Rosier P, Ulmsten U, van Kerrebroeck P, Victor A, Wein A (2002) The standardisation of terminology of lower urinary tract function: report from the Standardisation Sub-committee of the International Continence Society. *Neurourol Urodyn* **21**(2):167–78.

Andersson KE (2003) Storage and voiding symptoms: pathophysiologic aspects. *Urology* **62**(5 Suppl 2): 3–10.

Anger JT, Saigal CS, Wang M, Yano EM (2008) Urologic disease burden in the United States: veteran users of Department of Veterans Affairs healthcare. *Urology.* **72**(1): 37–41.

Berry SJ, Coffey DS, Ewing LL (1984) The development of human benign prostatic hyperplasia with age. *J Urol* **132**(3): 474–9.

Brown JA, Wilson TM (1997) Benign prostatic hyperplasia requiring transurethral resection of the prostate in a 60-year-old male-to-female transsexual. *Br J Urol* **80**: 956.

Casella R, Bubendorf L, Schaefer DJ, Bachmann A, Gasser TC., Sulser T (2005) Does the prostate really need androgens to grow? Transurethral resection of the prostate in a male-to-female transsexual 25 Years after sex-changing operation. *Urol Int* **75**: 288–90.

Coyne KS, Sexton CC, Thompson CL, Milsom I, Irwin D, Kopp ZS, Chapple CR, Kaplan S, Tubaro A, Aiyer LP, Wein AJ (2009) The prevalence of lower urinary tract symptoms (LUTS) in the USA, the UK and Sweden: results from the Epidemiology of LUTS (EpiLUTS) study. *BJU Int.* **104**(3): 352–60.

Fitzpatrick JM (2006) The natural history of benign prostatic hyperplasia. *BJU Int* **97**(2): 3–6.

Irwin DE, Milsom I, Hunskaar S, Reilly K, Kopp Z, Herschorn S, Coyne K, Kelleher C, Hampel C, Artibani W, Abrams P (2006) Population-based survey of urinary incontinence, overactive bladder, and other lower urinary tract symptoms in five countries: results of the EPIC study. *Eur Urol* **50**(6): 1306–14.

Jacobsen SJ, Girman CJ, Lieber MM (2001) Natural history of benign prostatic hyperplasia. *Urology* **58**(6 Suppl 1): 5–16.

Kaplan SA, Roehrborn CG, Chapple CR, Rosen RC, Irwin DE, Kopp Z, Aiyer LP, Mollon P (2009) Implications of recent epidemiology studies for the clinical management of lower urinary tract symptoms. *BJU Int* **103**(3): 48–57.

Kupelian V, Wei JT, O'Leary MP, Kusek JW, Litman HJ, Link CL, McKinlay JB (2006) BACH Survery Investigators. Prevalence of lower urinary tract symptoms and effect on quality of life in a racially and ethnically diverse random sample: the Boston Area Community Health (BACH) Survey. *Arch Intern Med* **166**(21): 2381–7.

Lee AJ, Garraway WM, Simpson RJ, Fisher W, King D (1998) The natural history of untreated lower urinary tract symptoms in middle-aged and elderly men over a period of five years. *Eur Urol* **34**: 325–32.

Lieber MM, Rhodes T, Jacobson DJ, McGree ME, Girman CJ, Jacobsen SJ, St Sauver JL (2009) Natural history of benign prostatic enlargement: long-term longitudinal population-based study of prostate volume doubling times. *BJU Int* Jul 7. [Epub ahead of print]

McNeal JE (1978) Origin and evolution of benign prostatic enlargement. *Invest Urol.* **15**(4): 340–5.

Roosen A, Chapple CR, Dmochowski RR, Fowler CJ, Gratzke C, Roehrborn CG, Stief CG, Andersson KE (2003) A Refocus on the Bladder as the Originator of Storage Lower Urinary Tract Symptoms: A Systematic Review of the Latest Literature. *Urology* **62**(5 Suppl 2): 3–10.

Naslund MJ, Gilsenan AW, Midkiff KD, Bown A, Wolford ET, Wang J (2007) Prevalence of lower urinary tract symptoms and prostate enlargement in the primary care setting. *Int J Clin Pract* **61**(9): 1437–45.

Temml C, Brossner C, Schatzl G, Ponholzer A, Knoepp L, Madersbacher S (2003) The natural history of lower urinary tract symptoms over five years. *Eur Urol* **43**: 374–80.

Wei JT, Calhoun E, Jacobsen SJ (2005) Urologic diseases in America project: benign prostatic hyperplasia. *J Urol* **173**(4): 1256–61.

Chapter 3

Pathophysiology of BPH, symptoms, and symptom scores

Reg Bruskewitz

Key points

- Lower urinary tract symptoms (LUTS) reflect outlet obstruction and irritative symptoms
- Benign prostatic hyperplasia (BPH) is a histological diagnosis and not a "disease".
- Prostatic enlargement is not closely correlated with the degree of obstruction to urine flow or to the presence of LUTS
- Over active bladder is common in many patients with BPH and LUTS.

Benign prostatic hyperplasia (BPH) is ubiquitous in aging males. This non malignant growth of epithelial and stromal tissue may physically impinge on the urethral lumen, causing obstruction to the flow of urine. The hyperplasia is not uniform and is often nodular and diffusely hyperplastic and located in the transition zone of the prostate directly adjacent to the urethral lumen.

- Enlargement may develop to varying degrees but is not closely correlated with the degree of obstruction to urine flow or to the presence of lower urinary tract symptoms (LUTS). Because of the immediate proximity of the prostate to the bladder base and bladder neck, interaction between the prostate and bladder, which is poorly understood but probably neurological to some degree, occurs and may result symptoms related to bladder dysfunction may be present as well.
- Overactive bladder and overactive bladder symptoms are present in many men with BPH. This overactive bladder complex may return toward normal with surgical treatment of BPH.

The prevalence of BPH on a histopathological basis is age dependant and is estimated to be 60% by age 60 and 90% at age 85.

- Androgens are necessary for the development of BPH, and androgen withdrawl results in partial regression of BPH. Overall the role of androgens in BPH development is incompletely understood. Young males absent androgen do not develop BPH. The prostate and prostatic capsule is rich in smooth as well as striated muscle. Alpha 1α adrenergic innervation of the muscle is believed to result in increased muscle tone and may contribute to the development of LUTS.

- Prostatic inflammation is frequently found in the hyperplastic prostate as well. The cause of the commonly found inflammation is unclear, and may be associated with LUTS and may be amenable to BPH medical therapy. This inflammation is chronic and associated with lymphocytic infiltration of the glandular and stromal tissue; this is distinct from the acute inflammation associated with bacterial prostatic infection or urinary tract infection.

- As the prostate changes with age so does the urinary bladder. Hypertrophy of the detrusor muscle, trabeculation and bladder wall fibrosis and denervation and re-innervation have been identified as hallmarks of aging. Impairment in detrusor contractility and development of bladder over activity are age related changes which may interact with or be confused with LUTS related to BPH.

> While LUTS may result from bladder or prostatic changes, LUTS in older men **may not be secondary to bladder outlet obstruction**. In a study of older men with LUTS, 50% had no evidence of obstruction.

Not that many years ago LUTS was commonly referred to as prostatism. This term implied that symptoms originated from the prostate and tended to lead the clinician to too quickly conclude that the prostate was the source of the symptoms. LUTS to a lesser degree suffers from the same tendency. For example the symptom nocturia, perhaps the most annoying of LUTS, may be related to nocturnal polyuria from any of a host of conditions including cardiac dysfunction, medication, or adrenal dysfunction.

> So LUTS, like prostatism, does not necessarily have origin in the prostate, and may not have origin in the *lower* urinary tract.

Initial publications addressing the "prostatism" symptoms included the Boyarski Symptom Assessment which evaluated lower urinary tract symptoms but was not validated. It did not incorporate an assessment of the degree of bother resulting form symptoms. The Madsen and Iversen BPH symptom score was first described in 1983. This scoring system addressed obstructive and irritative symptoms and assigned unequal weight to the various symptoms based on the authors' preconceptions about the relative and unequal importance of each of the symptoms. These first two LUTS scoring schemes were not formally statistically validated.

3.1 American Urological Association BPH Symptom Index Questionnaire

- Under the auspices of the American Urological Association ad hoc Measurement Committee the American Urological Association Symptom Index (AUASI) was developed. This was developed by utilizing the symptoms of the above two symptoms assessments as well as that used in the Maine Medical Association evaluation. In addition questions from the literature and questions about symptom severity and frequency provided by the Measurement Committee members were administered to men with "clinical BPH" as well as younger men in their 30s to obtain a reproducible and clinically and statistically validated score. Subsequently a quality of life (QoL) question; "If you were to spend the rest of your life with your urinary condition just the way it is now, how would you feel about that?" The original six questions became a seven question symptom score with the addition of the QoL.

The following form may be used to calculate the AUA BPH Symptom Index Score.

	Never	Less than 1 time in 5	Less than half the time	About half the time	More than half the time	Almost always
1. Over the past month or so, how often have you had a sensation of not emptying your bladder completely after you finished urinating?	⊙	○	○	○	○	○
2. Over the past month or so, how often have you had to urinate again less than two hours after you finished urinating?	⊙	○	○	○	○	○

	Never	Less than 1 time in 5	Less than half the time	About half the time	More than half the time	Almost always
3. Over the past month or so, how often have you found you stopped and started again several times when you urinated?	⊙	○	○	○	○	○
4. Over the past month or so, how often have you found it difficult to postpone urination?	⊙	○	○	○	○	○
5. Over the past month or so, how often have you had a weak urinary stream?	⊙	○	○	○	○	○
6. Over the past month or so, how often have you had to push or strain to begin urination?	⊙	○	○	○	○	○
7. Over the last month, how many times did you usually get up to urinate from the time you went to bed at night until the time you got up in the morning?	⊙ Never	○ 1 time	○ 2 times	○ 3 times	○ 4 times	○ 5 times or more

- The International Prostate Symptom Score (IPSS) uses the same scheme and includes three storage symptoms (frequency, nocturia, urgency) and four voiding symptoms (feeling of incomplete emptying, intermittency, straining, and weak stream) along with a degree of bother question.

Internatonal Prostate Symptom Score (IPSS)

Patient Name:_____ Date of Birth:_____ Today's Date:_____

In the past month	Not at all	Less than 1 in 5 times	Less than half the time	About half the time	More than half the time	Almost always	Your Score
1. Incomplete Emptying How often have you a sensation of not emptying your bladder?	0	1	2	3	4	5	
2. Frequency How often you had to urinate less than every two hours?	0	1	2	3	4	5	
3. Intermittency How often have you found you stopped and started again several times when you urinated?	0	1	2	3	4	5	
4. Urgency How often have you found it difficult to postpone urination?	0	1	2	3	4	5	
5. Weak Stream How often have you had a weak urinary stream?	0	1	2	3	4	5	
6. Straining How often have you had to strain to start urination?	0	1	2	3	4	5	
	None	1 time	2 times	3 times	4 times	5 times	
7. Nocturia How many times did you typically get up at night to urinated?	0	1	2	3	4	5	
Total IPSS Score:							

Quality of life due to urinary symptoms	Delighted	Pleased	Mostly Satisfied	Mixed	Mostly Dissatisfied	Unhappy	Teriible
If you were to spend the rest of your life with your urinary condition the way it is now, how would you feel about that?	0	1	2	3	4	5	6

Urine Leakage (Incontinence)	No Leakage	Mild (A few drops a day, no pad use)	Mild (More than a few drops a day, 1–2 pad/day)	Moderate (3 or more pads per day)	Severe Leakage Problems
Circle one	0	1	2	3	4

Over Please →

- For both the AUA-SI and the IPSS, a score below 7 is usually associated with a low discomfort. Between 7 and 18 patients complaining moderate (relevant) voiding proteins and a score above 18 usually represents significant voiding complaints. Treatment is usually initiated with high AUA or IPSS scores.

The ICIQ-MLUTS assesses eight storage symptoms which includes five questions on varying types of incontinence including stress, urge and post micturition dribble, along with five voiding symptoms developed by adding hesitancy to those found in the AUASI/IPSS.

Bother is assessed on a linear scale. The **ICIQ-MLUTS** assesses LUTS which is more likely to be caused by detrusor dysfunction rather than the prostate alone.

Other symptoms such as dysuria and gross hematuria may be associated with BPH, but less frequently. These symptoms should be evaluated independently for additional causes.

The ICIQ-MLUTS Long Form is a patient completed questionnaire for evaluating male lower urinary tract symptoms and input on quality of life (QoL) in research and clinical practice. This questionnaire is a more in-depth assesment than the ICIQ-MLUTS. The ICIQ-MLUTS Long-Form provides a detailed summary of the level and impact of urinary symptoms and can facilitate patient-clinician discussions. The Questionnaire includes 23 items (Table 3.1).

Table 3.1 Question items of ICIQ		
Question items	Frequency	Weak stream history
	Nocturia	Strength of stream (picture item)
	Urgency	Intermittency
	Urge urinary incontinence	Dysuria
	Bladder pain	Incomplete emptying
	Stress urinary incontinence	Terminal dribbling
	Unexplained urinary incontinence	Post micturition dribble
	Hesitancy	Nocturnal enuresis
	Straining to start urination	Pad usage
	Straining to continue urination	Double micturition
	Urination position	Urinary retention
	Strength of stream	

The scoring system reached to 1–84. Overall score with greater values indicate increased symptom severity. Bother scale are not incorporated in the overall score but indicate impact of individual symptom for the patient.

Symptom inquiry should take into account the interaction of prostate and urinary bladder, and the interaction between the two. And consideration should be given to causes outside of the lower urinary tract and to the degree of bother emanating form the LUTY. Increasing data links the development of LUTS to sexual dysfunction, but that is beyond the scope of this discussion.

References

Abrams P, Chapple C, Khoury S, Roehrborn C, de la Rosette J (2009) Evaluation and Treatment of Lower Urinary Tract Symptoms in Older Men *J Urol* **181**: 1779–87.

Barry MJ, Fowler FJJ, O'Leary MP, Bruskewitz RC, Holtgrewe HL, Mebust WK, Cockett AT (1992) The American Urological Association symptom index for benign prostatic hyperplasia. The Measurement Committee of the American Urological Association *J Urol* **148**(5): 1549–57.

Barry MJ, Fowler FJJ, O'Leary MP, Bruskewitz RC, Holtgrewe HL, Mebust WK (1992) Correlation of the American Urological Association symptom index with self-administered versions of the Madsen-Iversen, Boyarsky and Maine Medical Assessment Program symptom indexes. Measurement Committee of the American Urological Association *J Urol* **148**(5): 1558–63.

Donovan J, Abrams P, Peters T, Kay H, Chapple C, de la Rosette J, Kondo A (1996) Psychometric Validity and Reliability of the ICSmale Questionnaire *BJU* **77**: 554–62.

Madsen FA, Bruskewitz RC (1995) Clinical manifestations of benign prostatic hyperplasia *Urol Clin North Am* **22**: 291–8.

McVary KT (2008) Medical Treatment of Lower Urinary Tract Symptoms Secondary to BPH. Therapeutic Insights. Publication of the American Medical Association, September.

Roehrborn CG, McConnell JD (2007) benign prostatic hyperplasia: etiology, pathophysiology, and natural history. In Campbell-Walsh *Urology* Vol 3 pp. 2727–65. 9th ed. Philadelphia: Saunders.

Chapter 4

BPH, PSA, and the risk of having prostate cancer (PCA)

Seife Hailemariam and Lukas Bubendorf

> **Key points**
>
> - Benign prostatic hyperplasia (BPH) is a common benign disorder of the prostate that, when advanced, results in varying degrees of urinary obstruction with lower urinary tract symptoms (LUTS)
> - The disease represents a nodular enlargement of the prostate mainly in the transition zone (TZ) caused by hyperplasia of both glandular and stromal components
> - It occurs only in individuals with intact testes indicating androgen dependency
> - Despite topographic and architectural similarities between PCA arising in TZ and atypical adenomatous hyperplasia (AAH) and BPH, there is no convincing evidence linking BPH or AAH to PCA.

4.1 Benign prostatic hyperplasia

Benign prostatic hyperplasia (BPH) is a benign fibromuscular and adenomatous overgrowth of the prostate gland. Symptoms are those of bladder outlet obstruction: weak stream, hesitancy, urinary frequency, urgency, nocturia, incomplete emptying, terminal dribbling, overflow or urge incontinence, and complete urinary retention. Diagnosis is based primarily on digital rectal examination (DRE) and symptoms; cystoscopy, transrectal ultrasonography, urodynamic, or other imaging studies may also be needed. The symptoms are referred to as lower urinary tract symptoms (LUTS).

The pathogenesis of BPH remains unclear. It is assumed that multiple age-related factors such as immunologic, hormonal, and neural mechanisms play a role.

Histologically BPH consists of overgrowth of the epithelium and fibromuscular tissue of the transitional zone and the periurethral area (Figure 4.1a–b). Overgrowth can be limited to the stroma or the acinar epithelium, or both. It manifests as nodules or diffuse enlargement of the TZ and periurethral tissue. As men get older the proportion of epithelium to stroma increases probably as a result of androgenic stimulation.

Non-symptomatic histological evidence of BPH can be identified in as many as 8% of men between the ages of 31 to 40. BPH with LUTS prevails in one fourth of men between the ages of 50 to 59, and the prevalence further increases with age.

Fig 4.1 Benign histological alterations of the prostate.
A) Whole mount section of a radical prostatectomy specimen showing pronounced nodular hyperplasia of the central zone including the transitional zone. B) BPH at higher magnification with nodular hyperplasia of glands and fibromuscular stroma. C) Atypical adenomatous hyperplasia (synonym: adenosis) with benign small prostate glands showing pseudo-invasion into the stroma at the periphery of the nodule. D) Prostate biopsy with proliferative inflammatory atrophy (PIA). Small crowded glands with organoid architectural pattern and mild inflammatory infiltrates.

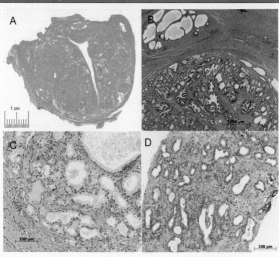

4.2 Associations between BPH and prostate cancer

Despite epidemiologic and anatomic associations between BPH and PCA, and the shared hormonal regulation, BPH is not considered as a precursor of PCA. Most PCA arise concomitantly with nodular hyperplasia, and approximately a quarter of all PCA originate in the transitional zone. This might suggest an etiologic association between BPH and PCA, at least in TZ PCA.

> BPH, even in case of very large dimensions, is not considered as a precursor of PCA.

- Atypical adenomatous hyperplasia (AAH; synonym: adenosis) has been discussed as a possible preneoplastic lesion of PCA in the TZ (Figure 4.1c). This hypothesis has remained controversial due to lack of clear evidence and molecular proof. Notably, the majority of PCA originates in the peripheral zone that is devoid of BPH. In an unselected population of men who where treated by open adenomectomy due to prostate enlargement (mean prostate volume 84 ml), Gratzke et al. found incidental carcinoma of the prostate in 28 of 902 patients (3.1%). It is important to mention that these included patients without preoperative investigations to exclude PCA because of advanced age.

Both BPH and PCA respond to androgen deprivation therapy. Like BPH, PCA is also strongly age-associated. The paradoxical increase in the prevalence of these two androgen-sensitive diseases at the time when the testosterone levels in the serum are decreasing suggests the involvement of other etiological factors. During the past few years, is has been recognized that estrogens and estrogen receptors might play an important role.

> While men's testosterone declines with age, the circulating levels of estradiol remain almost constant. This leads to a change in the estradiol/testosterone ratio that is temporally related to the onset of BPH and PCA (Figure 4.2).

Additionally, the effect of estrogens within the prostate is modulated by the presence of two different types of estrogen receptors (ER). ERα, which is mainly expressed in the stromal cells, is believed to mediate the adverse effects of estradiol including inflammation and carcinogenesis. In contrast, ERβ is expressed in the epithelial cells and seems to play a beneficial role being anti-proliferative and pro-apoptotic. Therefore, ERα antagonists and ERβ agonists are being discussed as interesting therapeutic strategies in PCA and BPH, respectively.

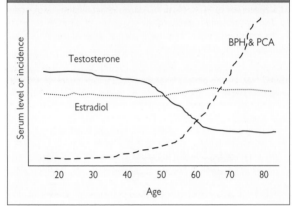

Fig 4.2 Testosterone levels continuously decrease with age, while the estrogen levels remain more or less unchanged. This results in an increasing estrogen-testosterone ratio that coincides with the increased incidence of BPH and prostate cancer

4.3 The role of metabolic syndrome and chronic inflammation

28

Metabolic syndrome and inflammation are other frequently related findings in both BPH and PCA. Some studies suggest that the metabolic syndrome is associated with BPH and PCA, and that hyperinsulinemia, dyslipidemia, elevated blood pressure, and obesity might be involved the pathogenesis of BPH and PCA. However, evidence for a causal relationship between metabolic syndrome and BPH and PCA remains weak.

It is known that longstanding chronic inflammation, which is associated with epithelial proliferation, can predispose to neoplastic transformation in different organs including liver, large bowel, urinary bladder, and gastric mucosa. Along this line, prostatic atrophy, which is associated with chronic inflammation and enhanced cell proliferation, has been suggested as a preneoplastic lesion in the prostate.

Proliferative inflammatory atrophy (PIA) designates foci of proliferative glandular epithelium with the morphological appearance of simple atrophy, or postatrophic hyperplasia, previously also referred to as postinflammatory atrophy, occurring in association with inflammation (Figure 4.1d).

PIA is preferentially found in the peripheral zone of the prostate – the origin of most PCA – rather than in the transitional zone. The pathogenesis of the common PIA lesion remains to be elucidated.

> One could speculate that chronic obstruction of the prostate ducts by BPH favours backpressure of secretion with consecutive PIA – thus indirectly linking BPH to PCA.

Other presumed causes of chronic inflammation of the prostate include a local estrogen effect and viral infections. It was hypothesized that subsequent loss of the detoxifying enzyme glutathione s-transferase pi (GSTpi) in PIA by gene promoter methylation favours accumulation of genetic damage through unopposed oxygen radicals, ultimately leading to PCA. Although this is an appealing hypothesis, there is so far no compelling clinical evidence that patients with PIA have in fact a higher risk of prostate cancer. Further studies are needed to elucidate the pathogenesis of PIA, and a possible link between PIA, chronic inflammation and PCA

4.4 **Prostatic specific antigen (PSA)**

PSA, also called kallikrein III, is a protein secreted by the epithelial cells of the prostate to liquefy the semen. In normal and hyperplastic prostate, PSA is uniformly present at the apical portion of the secretory epithelial cells of the prostatic glands. Since there is significant variation in PSA results among non-equimolar assays, the 90:10 ratio of complexed PSA to free PSA (the Stanford standard) was proposed as standardization; this became the basis for the PSA mass standards WHO 96/670 for tPSA and 96/668 for fPSA. Technical factors may also explain short-term PSA variability. Even the best of labs may report different results when they test the same blood sample twice, but these differences are usually small. In addition to changes that can be traced to specific causes, changes in the PSA can occur without evident explanation. There is always some variation between different equipments, and even the same type of machine may give slightly different results if used in different laboratories. Ideally, PSA testing is done in the same laboratory using the same equipment for individual patients.

Patients with elevated serum PSA levels are candidates for prostate biopsy in order to early detect prostate cancer. Although specific recommendations regarding PSA screening vary, there is general agreement that men should be informed about the potential risks and benefits of PSA screening before being tested.

In the past, most clinicians considered a PSA level below 4.0 ng/ml as normal. However, cancer was prevails in up to 15% of men with a PSA level at or below 4.0 ng/ml, and up to 15% of these men have are diagnosed with high-grade cancer. Among men with a PSA level between 4.1 and 9.9 ng/ml, biopsy reveals PCA in 25% to 35%, meaning that the biopsy is negative in 65 to 75% of these men.

> There is no specific threshold to separate a normal from an abnormal PSA level.

Various other factors, such as BPH and inflammation, can cause an elevated PSA level. Since PSA values can vary from laboratory to laboratory, a single abnormal PSA test result should be reconfirmed. Another valuable test for men with elevated PSA values is the analysis of free versus bound PSA. Most PSA in the blood is bound to other proteins. A smaller amount is unbound and called free PSA. Elevated free PSA is usually associated with benign prostate conditions (such as BPH, inflammation, or mechanical stress due to intensive bicycle riding). In contrast, a low ratio of bound versus free PSA (<25%) indicates a high risk of PCA.

References

Alcaraz A, Hammerer P, Tubaro A et al. (2009) Is there evidence of a relationship between benign prostatic hyperplasia and prostate cancer? Findings of a literature review *Urology* **55**: 864–75.

Bassett WW, Bettendorf DM, Lewis JM et al. (2009) Chronic periglandular inflammation on prostate needle biopsy does not increase the likelihood of cancer on subsequent biopsy *Urology* **73**: 845–9.

Cabelin MA, Te AE, Kaplan SA (2000) Benign prostatic hyperplasia: challenges for the new millennium *Curr Opin Urol* **10**: 301–6.

De Marzo AM, Platz EA, Sutcliffe S et al. (2007) Inflammation in prostate carcinogenesis *Nat Rev Cancer* **7**: 256–69. Review.

Ellem SJ, Risbridger GP (2007) Treating prostate cancer: a rationale for targeting local oestrogens *Nat Rev Cancer* **7**: 621–7. Review.

Leibovitch I, Mor Y (2005) The vicious cycling: bicycling related urogenital disorders *Eur Urol* **47**: 277–86. Review.

Gratzke C, Schlenker B, Seitz M et al. (2007) Complications and early postoperative outcome after open prostatectomy in patients with benign prostatic enlargement: results of a prospective multicenter study *J Urol* **177**: 1419–22.

Martin RM, Vatten L, Gunnell D et al. (2009) Components of the metabolic syndrome and risk of prostate cancer: the HUNT 2 cohort, Norway *Cancer Causes Control* **20**: 1181–92.

Mc Neal JE (1990) The pathobiology of nodular hyperplasia In: Bostwick DG, ed. *Pathology of the Prostate*, New York, NY: Churchill Livingstone: 31–6.

Ozden C, Ozdal OL, Urgacioglu G et al. (2007) The correlation between metabolic syndrome and prostatic growth in patients with benign prostatic hyperplasia *Eur Urol* **51**: 199–206.

Postma R, Schröder FH, van der Kwast TH (2005) Atrophy in prostate needle biopsy cores and its relationship to prostate cancer incidence in screened men *Urology* **65**: 745–9.

Prins GS, Korach KS (2008) The role of estrogens and estrogen receptors in normal prostate growth and disease *Steroids* **73**: 233–44. Review.

Smith DS, Humphrey PA, Catalona WJ (1997) The early detection of prostate carcinoma with prostate specific antigen: The Washington University experience *Cancer* **80**: 1853–6.

Thompson IM, Pauler DK, Goodman PJ et al. (2004) Prevalence of prostate cancer among men with a prostate specific antigen level < or = 4.0 ng per milliliter *N Engl J Med* **350**: 2239–46.

Vignati G, Giovanelli L (2007) Standardization of PSA measures: a reappraisal and an experience with WHO calibration of Beckman Coulter Access Hybritech total and free PSA *Int J Biol Markers* **22**: 295–301.

Chapter 5

Erectile dysfunction associated with LUTS and BPH

Thomas C. Gasser

> **Key points**
> - There is increasing evidence for an association between BPH/LUTS and ED
> - The adverse effects of medical treatment for BPH/LUTS on sexual function must be considered
> - Phospodiesterase—five inhibitors might play a future role in the treatment of BPH/LUTS.

According to the Massachusetts male aging study up to 52% of men between the age of 40 and 70 experience some kind of erectile dysfunction (ED) (Feldman et al., 1994). By the same token there is a clear increase of lower urinary tract symptoms (LUTS) due benign prostatic hyperplasia (BPH) with higher age.

> There is as a clear age dependence as the number of complete impotence tripled from 5.1% at the age of 40 to 15% at the age of 70.

For decades, ED and BPH/LUTS were considered to occur coincidentally in the same age group, but not directly related to each other. Recent studies, however, suggested an association between BPH/LUTS and sexual function. It appears that a significantly enlarged prostate has a downward effect not only on voiding but also on sexual function, mainly erection and ejaculation.

In a study of 1,274 men with LUTS, 55% with mild symptoms reported ED and 70% of those with severe symptoms (Vallancien et al., 2003). Moreover, reduced ejaculation were found in more than 50% and pain or discomfort during ejaculation in 7% to 31%.

> Every man's sexual function should be evaluated if he presents with LUTS.

One large, multinational survey in the USA and six European countries included more than 12,000 patients between the age of 50 and 80 (Rosen et al., 2003). A high 90% of the responders reported they had LUTS and 83% were sexually active. However, almost 49% suffered from ED. ED was significantly more common in men with BPH/LUTS. Taking into account age and comorbidities, erectile problems were clearly related to the severity of the voiding problems.

- A comprehensive review of the literature concluded that there was an association between BPH/LUTS and ED (McVary, 2005). However, based on the published epidemiological studies a causal relation could not be established. It was suggested that evaluating men with BPH/LUTS should include assessment of sexual function.
- Recent results from a BPH registry of almost 7,000 men provided additional evidence of the link between BPH/LUTS and ED (Rosen et al., 2009). Additionally, the authors focused on side effects of drugs commonly used to treat BPH/LUTS.

> There was a significant association between ED and ejaculatory disorders and α-blockers and 5-reductase inhibitors (5ARI).

Non-superselective AB (e.g. alfuzosin) were associated with better sexual function than superselective AB (e.g. tamsulosin), 5ARIs (e.g. finasteride) or the combination of both.

If a correlation between LUTS and ED is suspected one wonders if treatment of one might improve the other. As we have seen, medication used for BPH/LUTS at best has no effect on erectile function, but often does impair sexual function. Anecdotally however, some patients report on improved erectile function after successful surgical treatment of BPH, but the literature is sparse.

- A survey of the current literature found that several studies suggested a possible role of the nitric oxide/cGMP signalling pathway in the regulation of the prostate tone, which is in support of clinical observations (Roumeguere et al., 2009). Theoretically, phosphodiesterase-5-inhibitors (PDE-5) might have a beneficial effect on symptoms caused by prostatic enlargement. As a consequence, there was growing interest in the effect of PDE-5 inhibitors such as sildenafil and others on BPH/LUTS.

In 2007, a randomized, double-blind placebo controlled trial of 369 patients more than 45 years old treated with sildenafil with an open label extension was published (McVary et al., 2007). While there was a clear and expected improvement of erectile function in the sildenafil group it was also shown that sildenafil improved BPH/LUTS. In a dose finding study of 1058 men treated with tadalafil for BPH/LUTS a significant improvement of LUTS was found for 5, 10 and 20 mg (Roehrborn et al., 2008). However, no improvement of urine flow was noted.

• In a prospective, placebo controlled trial of twice daily vardenafil improvement of LUTS, erectile function and quality of life were found (Stief et al., 2008). Also in this study, no improvement of urine flow or postvoid residual urine was found. In a pilot study of 62 men, the combination of alfuzosin and sildenafil was superior to the monotherapy of either drug to improve both voiding and sexual dysfunction in men with LUTS suggestive of BPH (Kaplan et al., 2007). All these studies suggested a possible benefit of PDE-5 inhibitors on BPH/LUTS. However, larger, comparative, multicenter, non-industry sponsored trials with a longer follow-up are lacking.

In conclusion, there is increasing evidence for an association between BPH/LUTS and sexual dysfunction, mainly ED. However, further studies are needed to elucidate the pathophysiological background of these findings. Nevertheless, all patients presenting for BPH/LUTS should be assed as to their erectile function. Patients on medical treatment with α-blockers or 5ARI should be advised on possible side effects of these drugs on erectile function. Some patients with BPH/LUTS may benefit from PDE–5 inhibitors alone or in combination with AB. However, before such a treatment can generally be recommended, more studies are needed.

35

References

Feldman HA et al. (1994) Impotence and its medical and psychosocial correlates: Results of the Massachusetts male aging study *J Urol* **151**: 54–61.

Kaplan SA et al. (2007) Combination of alfuzosin and sildenafil is superior to monotherapy in treating lower urinary tract symptoms and erectile dysfunction *Eur Urol* **51**: 1717–23.

McVary KT (2005) Erectile dysfunction and lower urinary tract symptoms secondary to BPH *European Urology* **47**: 838–45.

McVary KT et al. (2007) Sildenafil citrate improves erectile function: a randomised double-blind trial with open-label extension *Int J Clin Pract* **61**: 1843–9.

Roehrborn, CG et al. (2008) Tadalafil administered once daily for lower urinary tract symptoms secondary to benign prostatic hyperplasia: A dose finding study *J Urol* **180**: 1228–34.

Rosen R et al. (2003) Lower urinary tract symptoms and male sexual dysfunction: The multinational survey of the aging male (MSAM-7) *European Urology* **44**: 637–49.

Vallancien G et al. (2003) Sexual dysfunction in 1,274 European men suffering from lower urinary tract symptoms *J Urol* **169**: 2257–61.

Rosen R et al. (2009) Association of sexual dysfunction with lower urinary tract symptoms of BPH and BPH medical therapies: Results from the BPH Registry *Urology* **73**: 562–6.

Roumeguère T et al. (2009) Is there a rationale for the chronic use of phosphodiesterase-5 inhibitors for lower urinary tract symptoms secondary to benign prostatic hyperplasia? *BJU Int.* **104**: 511–7.

Stief CG et al. (2008) A randomised, placebo-controlled study to assess the efficacy of twice-daily vardenafil in the treatment of lower urinary tract symptoms secondary to benign prostatic hyperplasia *Eur Urol.* **53**: 1236–44.

Chapter 6

OAB, LUTS, and BPH—a paradigm shift

Alexander Roosen

Key points

- "Overactive bladder" is a merely clinical diagnosis, comprising urgency, with or without urge incontinence (OAB-wet and OAB-dry), and either or both frequency and nocturia
- "Detrusor overactivity" (DO) is a urodynamic finding which may or may not underlay OAB, and has two types: phasic and terminal DO, the latter usually being of neurogenic origin
- "LUTS" comprise storage/OAB symptoms, voiding symptoms, and postmicturition symptoms. They equally affect men and women and are rather age- than gender-related
- In female OAB, antimuscarinics should be applied for 6–12 weeks before commencing invasive diagnostics. In the male, α_1-receptor antagonists should first be tried alone, followed by a combination with antimuscarinics.

6.1 Terminology

The symptomatic response of the lower urinary tract on different pathologies is rather uniform, the bladder therefore being referred to as an "unreliable witness".

Urinary symptoms in male patients with an enlarged prostate have traditionally been thought to originate from the prostate rather than from the bladder, whilst same symptoms in women have generally been attributed to bladder dysfunction. Thus, medical treatment of men with urinary symptoms usually targets the prostate, ignoring the bladder as possible site of origin.

The term "Lower Urinary Tract Symptoms" ("LUTS") was coined some 15 years ago to dissociate urinary symptoms from prostatic pathology. LUTS comprise voiding symptoms, postmicturition symptoms and storage symptoms which are also described by the term "overactive bladder" (OAB), as defined by the International Continence Society committee 2002 (Abrams et al., 2002) see also Chapters 1 and 2.

> The symptoms of an overactive bladder (OAB) are urgency, with or without urge incontinence (OAB-wet and OAB-dry), usually with frequency and nocturia

Urgency incontinence is the complaint of involuntary leakage accompanied by or immediately preceded by urgency. Urgency is the complaint of a sudden compelling desire to pass urine which is difficult to defer. Frequency is the complaint by the patient who considers that he/she voids too often by day. Nocturia is the complaint that the individual has to wake at night one or more times to void.

By contrast, detrusor overactivity (DO) is a merely urodynamic finding which may or may not underly OAB. It is characterized by involuntary detrusor contractions during the filling phase which may be spontaneous or provoked. The International Continence Society 2002 report describes two types:

- Phasic detrusor overactivity is defined by its characteristic waveform and may or may not lead to urinary incontinence
- Terminal detrusor overactivity is defined as a single involuntary detrusor contraction occurring at cystometric capacity, which cannot be suppressed, and causes incontinence.

Voiding symptoms may often be related to bladder outlet obstruction (BOO), as a result of benign prostatic obstruction (BPO), and are characterized by increased detrusor pressure and reduced urinary flow rate. BPO is regularly associated with benign prostatic enlargement (BPE), whereas the term benign prostatic hyperplasia (BPH) should be reserved for those cases in which hyperplastic tissue changes in the prostate are pathologically confirmed.

However, the relationship between voiding symptoms and urodynamic markers of prostatic conditions is as weak as is the relationship between OAB and DO (Chatelain, 2000).

6.2 **Epidemiology of OAB**

Voiding symptoms have been shown to be the most common LUTS in men, however, women also commonly present with voiding symptoms.

On the other hand, four of the five most bothersome LUTS in men are storage (OAB) symptoms. Prostatic pathology and co-existing OAB symptoms are not always causally related, and many men with OAB symptoms do not have BOO. However, OAB symptoms are highly prevalent in men: according to two telephone interview-based prevalence studies, they affect 16% of men and women in Europe and the US, with a striking age-related increase in both sexes, starting around the age of 40. Milsom et al. found a prevalence of OAB of 42 % in men older than 75 years.

- The latest international population-based survey, the EPIC study, confirmed these findings, i.e. OAB was equally common in men (11%) and women (13%) and storage, voiding, and postmicturition symptoms showed a similar distribution in both sexes. These data demonstrate that storage symptoms are not sex specific and that the prostate is often not the underlying cause of LUTS in men. They rather infer that LUTS are age-related and prevalent in both male and female patients, with a similar distribution of storage and voiding symptoms. However, although men and women had the same prevalence of OAB overall (16.0% and 16.9%, respectively), men were shown to have a higher prevalence of "OAB dry" (13.4% as opposed to 7.6% in women) and women had a higher prevalence of "OAB wet" (9.3% as opposed to 2.6% in men)

6.3 **Pathophysiology of OAB**

In keeping with the clinical notion that LUTS, and in particular OAB, are only poorly correlated with distinctive urodynamical findings, the up-to-date prevailing theories regarding the development of OAB are based on intrinsic bladder dysfunctions of multiple origin. Four theories, not mutually exclusive, have been put forth to account for bladder OAB:

1. The neurogenic hypothesis: reduced peripheral or central inhibition increases activation of the micturition reflex and contractions associated with the overactive bladder. This mechanism is the key principle in cases of neurogenic detrusor overactivity.

2. The myogenic hypothesis: changes to the excitability and coupling of smooth muscle cells with other myocytes or interstitial cells leads to the generation of uninhibited contractions. For example, bladder hypertrophy due to outlet obstruction may lead to so-called patchy denervation (German et al., 1995; Charlton et al., 1999; Drake et al, 2000; Mills et al., 2000). Smooth muscle cells deprived of their innervation show an up-regulation of membrane receptors and may have a higher excitability.

3. The urotheliogenic hypothesis: changes in the sensitivity and coupling of the suburothelial myofibroblast network lead to an enhancement of spontaneous detrusor activity.

4. The modular autonomous hypothesis: structures within the bladder wall coordinate to drive spontaneous contractions, which become enhanced in pathology.

6.4 Implications for diagnostic work-up and management

This paradigm shift in the clinical understanding of LUTS, namely that the bladder is the central organ in the pathogenesis, has a direct bearing on the assessment and management of LUTS.

As presence of the OAB syndrome is established on the basis of patient history, frequent flow charts, and questionnaires, it is common practice to employ conservative management (lifestyle interventions) and oral pharmacotherapy (antimuscarinics) without a urodynamic diagnosis. Trials of conservative and/or drug therapy for 6 to 12 weeks are regarded as reasonable before commencing invasive diagnostics.

The relevance of urodynamical testing remains controversial: detrusor overactivity has been shown to occur in 60% of asymptomatic women undergoing ambulatory urodynamics (Heslington and Hilton, 1996), and in a study of over 500 men with LUTS, only 53 % were found to have BOO. (Figure 6.1)

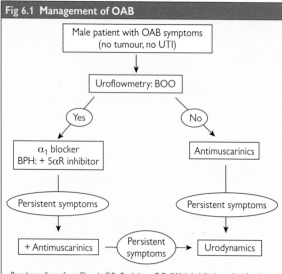

Fig 6.1 Management of OAB

Male patient with OAB symptoms (no tumour, no UTI)

↓

Uroflowmetry: BOO

Yes / No

α_1 blocker
BPH: + 5αR inhibitor

Antimuscarinics

Persistent symptoms

Persistent symptoms

+ Antimuscarinics → Persistent symptoms → Urodynamics

Based on a figure from Chapple C.R., Roehrborn C.G. (2006) A shifted paradigm for the further understanding, evaluation, and treatment of lower urinary tract symptoms in men: focus on the bladder Eur Urol **49**: 651–8. Reproduced with permission.

In the male, Chapple and Roehrborn propose a treatment plan based on the results of an assessment of overactive bladder symptoms, a physical examination, and a urinalysis:

- If bladder outlet obstruction is indicated by symptom assessment or uroflowmetry indicates bladder outlet obstruction, treatment should be commenced with an α_1-receptor antagonist
- If the prostatic gland is significantly hypertrophied, additional use of 5α-reductase inhibitor is recommended
- If the patient's condition does not show adequate improvement, antimuscarinics should be added for treatment of overactive bladder symptoms no matter if bladder outlet obstruction is present or not
- Urodynamic measurements should be performed in those cases where there is no symptom improvement with α_1-receptor antagonists, antimuscarinics, 5α-reductase inhibitors or combination therapy (Figure 6.2).

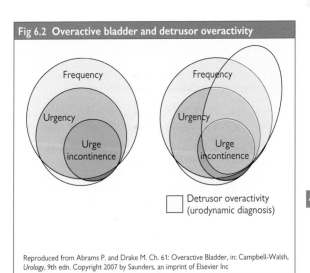

Fig 6.2 Overactive bladder and detrusor overactivity

Frequency

Urgency

Urge incontinence

Frequency

Urgency

Urge incontinence

☐ Detrusor overactivity (urodynamic diagnosis)

Reproduced from Abrams P. and Drake M. Ch. 61: Overactive Bladder, in: Campbell-Walsh, *Urology*, 9th edn. Copyright 2007 by Saunders, an imprint of Elsevier Inc

References

Abdel-Aziz KF, Lemack GE (2002) Overactive bladder in the male patient: bladder, outlet, or both? *Curr Urol Rep* **3**: 445–51.

Abrams P (1994) New words for old: lower urinary tract symptoms for "prostatism" *BMJ* 308: 929–30.

Abrams P, Cardozo L, Fall M, Griffiths D, Rosier P, Ulmsten U, Van Kerrebroeck P, Victor A, Wein A (2003) The standardisation of terminology in lower urinary tract function: report from the standardisation subcommittee of the International Continence Society *Urology* **61**: 37–49.

Brading AF (1997) A myogenic basis for the overactive bladder *Urology* **50**: 57–67; discussion 68–73.

Brading AF, Turner WH (1994) The unstable bladder: towards a common mechanism *Br J Urol* **73**: 3–8.

Chapple CR, Roehrborn CG (2006) A shifted paradigm for the further understanding, evaluation, and treatment of lower urinary tract symptoms in men: focus on the bladder *Eur Urol* **49**: 651–8.

Chapple CR, Wein AJ, Abrams P, Dmochowski RR, Giuliano F, Kaplan SA, McVary KT, Roehrborn CG (2008) Lower urinary tract symptoms revisited: a broader clinical perspective *Eur Urol* **54**: 563–9.

Eckhardt MD, van Venrooij GE, Boon TA (2001) Symptoms, prostate volume, and urodynamic findings in elderly male volunteers without and with LUTS and in patients with LUTS suggestive of benign prostatic hyperplasia *Urology* **58**: 966–71.

de Groat WC (1997) A neurologic basis for the overactive bladder *Urology* **50**: 36–52; discussion 53–6.

Drake MJ, Mills IW, Gillespie JI (2001) Model of peripheral autonomous modules and a myovesical plexus in normal and overactive bladder function *Lancet* **358**: 401–3.

Hyman MJ, Groutz A, Blaivas JG (2001) Detrusor instability in men: correlation of lower urinary tract symptoms with urodynamic findings *J Urol* **166**: 550–2; discussion 553.

Irwin DE, Milsom I, Hunskaar S, Reilly K, Kopp Z, Herschorn S, Coyne K, Kelleher C, Hampel C, Artibani W, Abrams P (2006) Population-based survey of urinary incontinence, overactive bladder, and other lower urinary tract symptoms in five countries: results of the EPIC study *Eur Urol* **50**: 1306–14; discussion 1314–5.

Kanai A, Roppolo J, Ikeda Y, Zabbarova I, Tai C, Birder L, Griffiths D, de Groat W, Fry C (2007) Origin of spontaneous activity in neonatal and adult rat bladders and its enhancement by stretch and muscarinic agonists *Am J Physiol Renal Physiol* **292**: F1065–72.

Milsom I, Abrams P, Cardozo L, Roberts RG, Thuroff J, Wein AJ (2001) How widespread are the symptoms of an overactive bladder and how are they managed? A population-based prevalence study *BJU Int* **87**: 760–6.

Stewart WF, Van Rooyen JB, Cundiff GW, Abrams P, Herzog AR, Corey R, Hunt TL, Wein AJ (2003) Prevalence and burden of overactive bladder in the United States *World J Urol* **20**: 327–36.

Temml C, Heidler S, Ponholzer A, Madersbacher S (2005) Prevalence of the overactive bladder syndrome by applying the International Continence Society definition *Eur Urol* **48**: 622–7.

Chapter 7

Bladder outflow obstruction, urodynamic studies and BPH

Julia Heinzelbecker and Maurice Stephan Michel

Key points

- The term bladder outflow/outlet obstruction (BOO) is an urodynamical diagnosis
- Only 50% of patients with BOO have prostatic enlargement
- Bladder outlet obstruction is always associated with changes in the bladder wall
- The impact of urodynamic studies in the evaluation of men with prostatic enlargement remains controversial.

7.1 Definition and etiology

The urodynamical diagnosis of bladder outflow obstruction (BOO) is usually caused by the enlargement of the prostate gland. BOO results in only approximately half of the patients with prostatic enlargement/growth (BPE). BOO due to prostatic enlargement/ growth is usually based on histological BPH. Even after urological and histological (e.g. prostate core biopsy) evaluation one can name it "benign prostatic obstruction (BPO)" (Adams, 1994).

BPH = benign prostatic hyperplasia – after histological evaluation
BPE = benign prostatic enlargement – prostate growth
BOO = bladder outflow obstruction – after urodynamical evaluation
BPO = benign prostatic obstruction – after histological and urodynamical evaluation

Evident BOO is always associated with changes in the bladder wall, i.e. muscle cell hypertrophy, elongation of cell or nucleus and infiltration of connective tissue between muscle cells. The impact of urodynamic studies in the evaluation of men with BPO remains controversial.

7.2 Assessment

Several methods exist to examine the degree of BOO. These include non invasive and urodynamic methods. Furthermore validated symptom questionnaires include beside irritative scores also obstructive scores.

7.2.1 Non-invasive methods

Non-invasive assesment methods are:

- Uroflowmetry
- Peak flow rate (Qmax) is correlated to volume voided. The objective value of uroflowmetry remains controversial so it only serves as an indirect measure of obstruction
- Postvoidal residual urine (PVR)
- Differing classifications exist. Attention has to be paid as results can reflect BOO **or** detrusor underactivity (DUA)
- Urodynamic methods
- Urodynamically the detrusor pressure (pdet) at maximum flow (Qmax) describes the grade of BOO.

Several nomograms exist to illustrate this coherence:

- Abrams-Griffiths nomogram
- Linear passive urethral resistance relation (LinPURR)
- Urethral resistance factor.
- Validated symptom questionnaires
  - IPSS (International Prostatic Symptome Score)
  - AUA-SI (American Urological Association symptom index)

These consist of irritative and obstructive scores and are designed for the evaluation of LUTS. However, 20 to 30% of men with LUTS due to BPH do not show BOO. Only little or no correlation between LUTS and BOO exist (de la Rosette et al., 1998).

Nowadays urodynamically received pressure/flow studies are considered the only objective method to detect BOO.

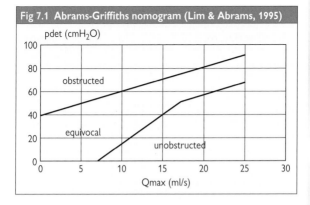

Fig 7.1 Abrams-Griffiths nomogram (Lim & Abrams, 1995)

7.3 **Urodynamic studies and benign prostatic obstruction (BPD)**

The role and benefit of urodynamic studies prior to BPO therapy still remain controversial. The following comprises an overview of urodynamic findings and their impact on treatment outcome.

1. Urodynamic results under medication therapy

   Common initial treatment of men with LUTS because of BPH comprises alpha-adrenergic receptor antagonists or 5-alpha reductase inhibitors.

2. Urodynamic results and outcome after surgical therapy

   It is often discussed if urodynamic studies prior to surgery can make a change in reduction of overall morbidity, financial savings and most important treatment outcome.

> There is consensus that patients with BPO have a higher success rate from deobstructive surgery than those without BPO (Javlé et al., 1998; Van Venrooij et al., 2002; Seki et al., 2006; Tanaka et al., 2006)

Nevertheless studies exist that point out that patients selected for surgery by symptoms only have a favourable outcome regardless of their urodynamic results before surgery and that in terms of quality of life (QoL). The QoL index remains improved in long-term follow up regardless of the preoperative urodynamic findings (Frimodt-Møller et al., 1984; Masumori et al., 2009).

3. Urodynamic detrusor overactivity and BOO

The prevalence of detrusor overactivity continuously rises with increasing BOO grade (Oelke et al., 2008). In case of pre-existing DO patients had a significant better outcome according to persistent urgency, frequency and incontinence in case of BOO than in case of mere LUTS without BOO (Robertson et al., 1996).

> International continence society (ISC) definition: "urodynamic observation characterized by involuntary detrusor contractions during the filling phase which may be spontaneous or provoked" (Abrams et al., 2002).

In BPO patients presenting with detrusor overactivity, deobstructive surgery provides the opportunity to reverse bladder wall changes and detrusor overactivity. A combination of alpha-adrenergic receptor antagonists and muscarine receptor antagonists displays an alternative especially in patients inadequate for surgery (Athanasopoulos et al., 2003; Lee et al., 2004).

Nevertheless differential diagnoses as neurologic disorders have to be considered.

- Prevalence of detrusor overactivity rises with grade of BOO
- In case of BOO + detrusor overactivity deobstructive surgery is indicated
- Combinative medication therapy is possible
- Patients with detrusor overactivity in absence of BOO need further evaluation.

4. Urodynamic detrusor underactivity and BOO

In patients complaining for LUTS it is not possible to differentiate between detrusor underactivity and BOO neither by symptoms nor by flow rate. Thus only by urodynamic studies detrusor underactivity can be diagnosed.

> ICS definition: "a contraction of reduced strength and/or duration, resulting in prolonged bladder emptying and/or failure to achieve complete bladder emptying within a normal time span".

There is no evidence to suggest that detrusor contractility diminishes with long-term BOO and furthermore that deobstructive surgery does not improve detrusor contractility (Al-Hayek et al., 2004; Thomas et al., 2004). But as other studies show improved symptoms, QoL and PVR after deobstructive surgery, its benefit in patients with detrusor underactivity finally remains unclear (Han et al., 2008).

Moreover the co-existance of BOO and underactive detrusor has to be considered. In this condition the detrusor may fail to rise sufficiently and the BOO may be misdiagnosed. However, benefit of surgery remains controversial, as those patients always need to have an individual approach.

An urodynamic analysis does not appear to be necessary in the majority of men with voiding symptoms secondary to BPH. However, those men with neurologic disorders and those with persistent or recurrent symptoms following deobstructive prostate surgery represent a more complex patient population. In these patients a more thorough evaluation has to be performed.

Furthermore, in investigational clinical trials accurate urodynamic settings are mandatory.

When to perform urodynamic studies?

- In men with neurologic disorders
- In men with persistent or recurrent symptoms after deobstructive surgery
- In investigational clinical trials.

References

Abrams P (1994) New words for old: lower urinary tract symptoms for "prostatism" *BMJ* **308**: 929–30.

Abrams P, Cardozo L, Fall M et al. (2002) The standardisation of terminology of lower urinary tract function: report from the Standardisation Sub-committee of the International Continence Society *Neurourol Urodyn* **21**: 167–78.

Al-Hayek S, Thomas A, Abrams P (2004) Natural history of detrusor contractility—minimum ten-year urodynamic follow-up in men with bladder outlet obstruction and those with detrusor *Scand J Urol Nephrol Suppl* **215**: 101–8.

Athanasopoulos A, Gyftopoulos K, Giannitsas K et al. (2003) Combination treatment with an alpha-blocker plus an anticholinergic for bladder outlet obstruction: a prospective, randomized, controlled study *J Urol* **169**: 2253–6.

de la Rosette JJ, Witjes WP, Schäfer W et al. (1998) Relationships between lower urinary tract symptoms and bladder outlet obstruction: results from the ICS-"BPH" study *Neurourol Urodyn* **17**: 99–108.

Frimodt-Møller PC, Jensen KM, Iversen P, Madsen PO, Bruskewitz RC (1984) Analysis of presenting symptoms in prostatism *J Urol* **132**: 272–6.

Han DH, Jeong YS, Choo MS, Lee KS (2008) The efficacy of transurethral resection of the prostate in the patients with weak bladder contractility index *Urology* **71**: 657–61.

Javlé P, Jenkins SA, Machin DG, Parsons KF (1998) Grading of benign prostatic obstruction can predict the outcome of transurethral prostatectomy *J Urol* **160**: 1713–7.

Lee JY, Kim HW, Lee SJ et al. (2004) Comparison of doxazosin with or without tolterodine in men with symptomatic bladder outlet obstruction and an overactive bladder *BJU Int* **94**: 817–20.

Lim CS, Abrams P (1995) The Abrams-Griffiths nomogram *World J Urol* **13**: 34–9.

Masumori N, Furuya R, Tanaka Y et al. (2009) The 12-year symptomatic outcome of transurethral resection of the prostate for patients with lower urinary tract symptoms suggestive of benign prostatic obstruction compared to the urodynamic findings before surgery *BJU Int* Oct 26, Epub ahead of print

Oelke M, Baard J, Wijkstra H et al. (2008) Age and bladder outlet obstruction are independently associated with detrusor overactivity in patients with benign prostatic hyperplasia *Eur Urol* **54**: 419–26.

Robertson AS, Griffiths C, Neal DE (1996) Conventional urodynamics and ambulatory monitoring in the definition and management of bladder outflow obstruction *J Urol* **155**: 506–11.

Seki N, Takei M, Yamaguchi A, Naito S (2006) Analysis of prognostic factors regarding the outcome after a transurethral resection for symptomatic benign prostatic enlargement *Neurourol Urodyn* **25**: 428–32.

Tanaka Y, Masumori N, Itoh N et al. (2006) Is the short-term outcome of transurethral resection of the prostate affected by preoperative degree of bladder outlet obstruction, status of detrusor contractility or detrusor overactivity? **13**: 1398–404.

Thomas AW, Cannon A, Bartlett E, Ellis-Jones J, Abrams P (2004) The natural history of lower urinary tract dysfunction in men: the influence of detrusor underactivity on the outcome after transurethral resection of the prostate with a minimum 10-year urodynamic follow-up *BJU Int* **93**: 745–50.

Van Venrooij GE, Van Melick HH, Eckhardt MD, Boon TA (2002) Correlations of urodynamic changes with changes in symptoms and well-being after transurethral resection of the prostate *J Urol* **168**: 605–9.

Chapter 8

Aging men and LUTS

Stephan Degener and Michael J. Mathers

> ### Key points
> - LUTS is a common problem in aging men even in absence of BPH with negative impact on quality of life
> - Age-related changes, e.g. in the bladder, the kidney or the testosterone level can cause LUTS
> - Neurological, cardiovascular or endocrine diseases as well as malignancy and infections can evoke LUTS
> - LUTS has negative impact on patients' QoL and healthcare system costs, therefore its treatment needs a more integrative approach.

Lower urinary tract symptoms (LUTS) are a major problem for the elderly. The prevalence of both BPH and LUTS increase with age: At least 50% of men have pathological benign prostatic hyperplasia (BPH) at age 51–60 years but close to 90% of the male population by the age of 80. The prevalence of LUTS increases from 10.5% at age 30–39 years to 25.5% at age 70–79 years.

Traditionally, lower urinary tract symptoms in men have been termed "prostatism" because of their close relation. Meanwhile, there is the cognition that bladder dysfunction may also cause LUTS as well as a wide spectrum of physical and mental disabilities, co-morbidities, (multi-)medication or even "just" age-related non-pathological changes.

Therefore, the diagnosis of LUTS requires a more integrative approach with a detailed clinical evaluation—voiding symptoms as well as the general physical, mental, and medical condition. Although it is often difficult to determine the causal factor and mostly the genesis of LUTS is multifactorial.

8.1 Age-related changes in elderly related to LUTS

Naturally, age-related BPH is an important factor in the pathophysiology of LUTS. It affects most men and causes infravesical obstruction in almost 50% of them. But even in the absence of diseases, the lower urinary tract changes with age.

- Overactive Bladder (OAB) is a complex of symptoms defined as urgency with or without urge urinary incontinence (63% are continent) usually with increased daytime frequency and nocturia in the absence of pathologic or metabolic causes (neurogenic and myogenic factors and urothelial dysfunction are discussed in the aetiology)

- Urodynamicly, OAB is characterized by involuntary detrusor contractions during bladder filling despite the patient's attempt to suppress them (detrusor instability, irritable bladder, etc.). The prevalence of OAB in adults older than 75 years is 35% vs. 16% in general population. Antimuscarinic agents are first-line therapy at best in combination with behavioural therapy (bladder training), physiotherapy, electrotherapy or instrumental biofeedback. Botulinum is currently being investigated

- Impaired detrusor function can present in two ways: insufficiency in generating pressure or in contraction sustainability. Contractility values decrease from 30 W/m^2 in adolescence to about 12 W/m^2 (70 years) and fading contractions occur because a limited amount of energy available for bladder emptying. These findings are compatible with urodynamic abnormalities in elderly like detrusor contractility, bladder capacity, the ability to postpone voiding and decreased urinary flow with increasing age

- Nocturia (≥1 nightly awakening by urge to void) affects 45% of individuals over 50 years even in the absence of heart failure, renal disease or venous insufficiency. In the elderly about one half of total 24h urinary sodium is excreted during nighttime, resulting in larger nocturnal urine volumes. The reason exact is unknown

- Testosterone: Plasma levels decline with aging and coincide with the emergence of LUTS. The association of LUTS and erectile dysfunction (ED) is well-known. The pathogenetic relationship is not yet completely understood (probably a decrease of NOS/NO in the endothelium) and the role of sex hormone levels in LUTS is discussed controversially

- Immobility is one of the main handicaps in the elderly and should be considered in LUTS diagnostic. An elongated time to get up or to arrive the bathroom can simulate LUTS.

8.2 **Pathophysiologic conditions evoking LUTS**

Morbidity increases with aging and consequently the incidence of diseases evoking lower urinary tract symptoms (acute and chronic) increases:

- Transient problems: Transient factors for LUTS have been subsumed in the mnemonic trick DIAPPERS: delirium, infection, (atrophic vaginitis), pharmaceuticals, psychological factors, excess urine output, restricted mobility, and stool impaction

- Cerebrovascular accident: LUTS is common after stroke with detrusor overactivity as most common long-term expression. Generally sensation is intact thus the patient suffers from urgency (70%) with nocturia (76%) and daytime frequency (59%). Urgency is the most severe symptom. If the patient is not able to contract the sphincter voluntarily, urgency with incontinence results. In urodynamics, the most frequent findings are detrusor hyperreflexia (68%) and involuntary sphincter relaxation (36%). Urinary retention in acute stroke is infrequent (6%)

- Parkinson's disease: In addition to the motor skills, also the autonomic nervous system (ANS) is affected causing LUTS with nocturia, frequency and urgency being the most frequent. Studies show a prevalence of urinary disturbances in 38%–71%. Urodynamic evaluation most frequently shows detrusor overactivity but also hyporeflexia, areflexia or even normal function. The smooth sphincter is synergic. The pharmacological therapy of Parkinson's disease also has a positive effect on voiding dysfunctions. Attention should be paid to the differential diagnosis multiple system atrophy. An abnormal sphincter electromyography (EMG) indicates a multiple system atrophy

- Diabetes mellitus type II (DM): Diabetic cystopathy is a progressive condition that begins with the loss of viscerosensory innervation of the bladder parallel to the diabetic polyneuropathy. The exact incidence is uncertain: between 5–59% of diabetic patients report on voiding symptoms. Urodynamicly, it is mainly characterized by diminished bladder sensation, increased cystometric capacity but decreased bladder contractility resulting in impaired uroflow and increased post-void residual urine

- Dementia: Although the debut of inhibited detrusor contraction correlates with subcortical white matter lesions and the disease progress, studies have shown that impaired mobility is a stronger determinant of urinary incontinence than cognitive impairment. Many patients are still able to walk (with assistance) to the bathroom. There are neither reliably data on pharmacological nor on interventional therapies. Behaviour conditioning and micturition training adapted to the individual cognitive and physical skills also appear to be helpful too.

Furthermore, congestive heart failure, bladder cancer, prostate cancer, urinary tract infections, urethral stricture and bladder neck hypertrophy are known to cause LUTS identical to BPH.

The number of men achieving an old age increases and with it the incidence of LUTS. Older men often accept it as a normal part of growing older but it is well known that LUTS has negative a impact on quality of life, regardless of the underlying aetiology.

Furthermore, LUTS causes enormous costs for the health care system due to therapy costs and secondary costs such as LUTS forwards the patients' placement in nurseries or increases the risk of falls in older men.

References

Braun MH, Sommer F, Haupt G et al. (2003) Lower urinary tract symptoms and erectile dysfunction: co-morbidity or typical "Aging Male" symptoms? Results of the "Cologne Male Survey" *Eur Urol* **44**: 588–94.

Dubeau CE (2006) The aging lower urinary tract *J Urol* **175**: 11–15.

Gomes CM, Arap S, Trigo-Rocha FE (2004) Voiding dysfunction and urodynamic abnormalities in elderly patients *Rev Hosp Clin* **59**: 206–15.

Kaye M (2008) Aging, circadian weight change, and Nocturia *Nephron Physiol* **109**: 11–18.

Lepor H (2005) Pathophysiology of lower urinary tract symptoms in the aging male population *Rev Urol* **7**: 3–11.

Nordling J (2002) The aging bladder – a significant but underestimated role in the development of lower urinary tract symptoms *Exp Gerontol* **37**: 991–9.

Wein AJ (2007) Lower urinary tract dysfunction in neurologic injury and disease, in: *Campbell-Walsh Urology*, 9th ed, Saunders Elsevier, Philadelphia.

Chapter 9

Risk factors associated with BPH

Stavros Gravas

> **Key points**
>
> - The etiopathogenesis of BPH is still largely unresolved
> - The only clearly defined risk factors for BPH include age and the presence of circulating androgens
> - Epidemiologic data suggest that several factors including metabolic syndrome, sexual activity, alcohol intake, dietary factors seem to play a role as determinants of disease
> - Advancing age, increased prostate size, and higher serum PSA levels represent the most significant risk factors for the occurrence of acute urinary retention and need for surgery.

Benign prostatic hyperplasia is a progressive disease that is commonly associated with bothersome LUTS and might result in complications such as acute urinary retention and BPH-related surgery.

The term 'BPH' actually refers to a histological condition, namely the presence of stromal-glandular hyperplasia within the prostate gland. A standardized clinical definition of BPH is lacking, and the use of various different study designs in longitudinal studies hamper the determination of risk factors for development of clinical BPH.

There is an increasing understanding that male LUTS result from several pathophysiological conditions, but BPH has been recognized as a major contributing factor for LUTS in aging men.

9.1 Risk factors for development of BPH

The aetiopathogenesis of BPH is still largely unresolved and the only clearly defined risk factors for BPH include age and the presence of circulating androgens.

- Age has been shown to be a critical determinant of BPH since all studies reported a clear trend toward an increase in symptom scores and prostate volume (determined by transrectal ultrasound) with advancing age
- The incidence of BPH increases with age and it affects 50% of men of age 50 years or older, and increases to 90% in men age 80 years or older
- Androgens do not cause BPH, but the development of BPH requires the presence of testicular androgens during prostate development, puberty, and aging. Patients castrated prior to puberty or who are affected by a variety of genetic diseases that impair androgen action or production, do not usually develop BPH.

More recently, a growing body of evidence has demonstrated a strong and independent link between BPH/LUTS and other multiple factors that may influence the development of clinical disease. These include:

- *Genetics:* Family history of BPH has been reported as a risk factor for clinical BPH. Male relatives of men with early onset of BPH are at greater risk of being afflicted by the disorder. In addition, a variation in the incidence of BPH among different racial and ethnic subgroups has been reported a result of racial and ethnic differences in genetic factors related to androgen receptor CAG repeats, the androgen signalling pathway, and in the cellular composition of the prostate but also in diet and other lifestyle habits
- *Metabolic Syndrome:* This is a clinical constellation of metabolic abnormalities, including obesity, glucose intolerance, dyslipidemia and hypertension. Current evidence has consistently demonstrated strong associations of components of metabolic syndrome with an increased risk of BPH and LUTS. Factors including autonomic hyperactivity, hyperinsulinemia, inflammation, and obesity may play a role in the causes of both clinical entities
- *Diet:* Several studies have indicated that macronutrients and micronutrients may affect the risk of BPH and LUTS. Other studies have reported a direct association of polyunsaturated fatty acids with BPH. However, the precise role of dietary habits in the development of BPH has not been clearly defined
- *Alcohol consumption* has been reported to have a protective effect on BPH. This may be due to decrease plasma testosterone levels and production by alcohol

- *Physical activity:* Increased physical activity has been associated with a decreased risk of BPH and LUTS in several large cross-sectional studies. This suggests that exercise is a protective factor probably due to promotion of weight loss, enhancement of vascular flow, and normalization of serum lipid and lipoprotein concentrations. A recent meta-analysis confirmed that moderate to vigorous physical activity may reduce the risk of BPH or LUTS by as much as 25% relative to a sedentary lifestyle

- *Smoking:* Several studies suggest an inverse relationship between smoking and BPH probably due to appetite suppression and decreased adiposity. On the other hand, smoking is associated with an increased risk of metabolic syndrome. Therefore, the smoking/BPH relationship is likely to be weak

- *Sexual dysfunction:* Several large-scale epidemiological studies in men that sexual dysfunction and BPH are highly prevalent in aging men and are strongly linked independently of age and cardiovascular comorbidities.

Four theories supporting biological plausibility currently exist including the:

- nitric oxide synthase (NOS)/NO theory
- the autonomic hyperactivity and metabolic syndrome hypothesis
- the Rho-kinase activation/endothelin pathway; and
- pelvic atherosclerosis.

9.2 Risk factors to have surgery

The natural history of BPH may be observed from longitudinal population-based studies and from the placebo arms of controlled trials. In general, BPH is a chronic, complex disease that is progressive in many men. Analysis of the placebo arm of the Medical Therapy of Prostatic Symptoms (MTOPS) study showed that the rate of overall clinical progression of BPH events (defined as IPSS increase ≥4 points, acute urinary retention (AUR), urinary incontinence, renal insufficiency, or recurrent urinary tract infections) in the placebo group was 4.5 per 100 person-years, for a cumulative incidence of 17% among men who had follow-up data of at least 4 years.

Longitudinal data from the Veteran's Affairs study in the USA has demonstrated that 36% of men with BPH randomized to watchful waiting switched to invasive therapy within 5 years of enrolment.

The two most significant progression events are AUR and the need for BPH-related surgery. AUR results in prostatectomy in 24–42% of men in the UK and USA, and even patients who avoid surgery through a successful trial without catheter are subsequently at high risk of requiring surgery within a year. Although AUR and surgery are less common than overall symptomatic worsening, they are important progression events because of the financial, emotional and health-related implications and represent the major concerns of BPH patients. Rate of AUR was 0.6 events/100 person-years in the placebo group of the MTOPS trial whereas in terms of risk for invasive BPH therapy, the placebo group experienced 1.3 events/100 person-years.

A systematic review of the placebo arms of randomized trials of medical therapy for BPH tried to estimate rates of progression. Studies with a follow-up 12–48 months reported rates of surgery that varied from 1% to 10% whereas the rates of AUR were 0.4–6.6%; these rates tended to be worse with a longer follow-up. This remarkable variety in results may be explained by the differences and heterogeneity observed among the studies.

- Several risks factors at baseline were identified for disease progression from the placebo arm of the MTOPS such as:
  - prostate volume ≥31 ml,
  - PSA concentration ≥1.6 ng/ml,
  - Qmax ≤10.6 ml/s,
  - postvoid residual volume (PRV) ≥39 ml and
  - age ≥62 years.
- In the Olmsted County study, a strong age-related increase in the risk of BPH treatment over the 6 years of follow-up was reported (9 times the risk of any treatment, for men aged 70–79 vs men aged 40–49 years). The presence of moderate to severe LUTS (AUA SI >7), a decreased peak urinary flow (<12 mL/s), enlarged prostate volume (>30 mL), and an elevated serum PSA (> 1.4 ng/mL) were also found to be associated with a 4 times risk of BPH treatment (either medical or surgical)
- Similarly, a linear increase in the incidence of AUR and need for BPH-related surgery, with baseline serum PSA values was found in the in the Proscar Long-term Efficacy and Safety Study (PLESS®). The risk of BPH-related surgery increased from approximately 10% in men with a PSA level of <1 ng/mL to nearly 24% in men with a PSA level of >8 ng/mL, in the placebo arm with a follow-up of 4 years
- In the Alfuzosin 10 mg once daily Long-Term Efficacy And Safety Study (ALTESS) with a follow-up of 2 years, the risk of BPH-related surgery was driven by PSA values at baseline, the risk being five times greater for men with a PSA greater than 3.9 ng/ml (11.0%) compared to those with a PSA less than 2.3 ng/ml (2.1%). The risk of BPH-related surgery also tended to increase for those with severe LUTS at baseline (8.4% for severe LUTS vs 5.1% for moderate LUTS)

- In addition, there is increasing evidence that dynamic variables including symptom and PVR worsening serve as good predictors of AUR or BPH-related surgery in men with LUTS suggestive of BPH.

> Patients in the placebo group who did not develop AUR during the follow-up period had a stable PVR throughout the study, while those who subsequently developed AUR had a steady increase in PVR.

The relative importance of these risk factors as established in the absence of specific treatment may differ in a patient receiving treatment. To use these risk factors to predict progression will also require confirmation in an independent patient group.

9.3 **Risk factors to have recurrent BPH**

The patients' baseline variables influence their initial management (watchful waiting, medical treatment or surgical procedure) and subsequent improvement or worsening of LUTS influences further intervention. Recurrent BPH can be characterized as the progression of the disease despite an initial response to medical treatment. By far the most commonly used class of drugs for the treatment of bothersome LUTS associated with BPH is the alpha-adrenergic receptor blockers.

- The MTOPS study showed that doxazosin resulted in significant improvements in symptom scores versus placebo but doxazosin did not significantly reduced the risk of AUR and the need for BPH-related surgery.

Similarly, the ALTESS demonstrated that alfuzosin administered for 2 years achieved significant 30% reduction in LUTS deterioration but alfuzosin did not significantly reduce the risk of AUR and BPH-related surgery, compared to placebo. These data suggest that that in certain select patients, namely those with larger glands and likely higher serum PSA of combination treatment of an alpha-blocker with a 5-reductase inhibitor provides long-term superiority with regard to both symptom reduction and disease progression.

Based on the above described conditions and studies, advancing age, increased prostate size, higher baseline symptoms and higher serum PSA levels seem to predict treatment failure and represent the most possible risk factors for BPH recurrence. Clearly further work is needed to refine just who will and who will not benefit from the therapeutic options described above and which the risk factors for BPH recurrence are.

References

Emberton M, Cornel EB, Bassi PF et al. (2008) Benign prostatic hyperplasia as a progressive disease: a guide to the risk factors and options for medical management *Int J Clin Pract* **62**: 1076–86.

Fitzpatrick JM (2006) The natural history of benign prostatic hyperplasia *BJU Int* **97**(2): 3–6.

Kellogs Parsons J (2007) Modifiable risk factors for Benign Prostatic Hyperplasia and Lower Urinary Tract symptoms: New approaches to old problems *J Urol* **178**: 395–401.

Lepor H, Williford WO, Barry MJ et al. (1996) The efficacy of terazosin, finasteride, or both in benign prostatic hyperplasia. Veterans Affairs Cooperative Studies Benign Prostatic Hyperplasia Study Group *N Engl J Med*;**335**: 533–9.

McConnell JD, Bruskewitz R, Walsh P et al. (1998) The effect of finasteride on the risk of acute urinary retention and the need for surgical treatment among men with benign prostatic hyperplasia. Finasteride Long-Term Efficacy and Safety Study Group *N Engl J Med* **338**: 557–63.

McConnell JD, Roehrborn CG, Bautista OM et al. (2003) The long-term effect of doxazosin, finasteride, and combination therapy on the clinical progression of benign prostatic hyperplasia *N Engl J Med* **349**: 2387–98.

Moul S, McVary KT (2010) Lower urinary tract symptoms, obesity and the metabolic syndrome *Curr Opin Urol* **20**: 7–12.

Roehrborn CG (2008) BPH progression: concept and key learning from MTOPS, ALTESS, COMBAT, and ALF-ONE *BJU Int* **101**(S3): 17–21.

Rosen RC (2006) Update on the relationship between sexual dysfunction and lower urinary tract symptoms/benign prostatic hyperplasia *Curr Opin Urol* **16**: 11–19.

Roehrborn CG (2006) Alfuzosin 10 mg once daily prevents overall clinical progression of benign prostatic hyperplasia but not acute urinary retention: results of a 2-year placebo-controlled study *BJU Int* **97**: 734–41.

Roehrborn CG (2006) Definition of at-risk patients: baseline variables *BJU Int* **97**(2): 7–11.

Roehrborn CG, Siami P, Barkin J et al. (2008) The effects of dutasteride, tamsulosin and combination therapy on lower urinary tract symptoms in men with benign prostatic hyperplasia and prostatic enlargement: 2-year results from the CombAT study *J Urol* **179**: 616–21.

Chapter 10

Diagnosis and assessment of BPH: subjective parameters

Herbert Leyh

Key points

- Lower urinary tract symptoms (LUTS) may be the result of BPH
- The symptoms of BPH can be divided in obstructive and irritative symptoms
- More important than a single determination of symptoms is the dynamic process of symptom changes
- The correlation between the extent of symptoms and the prostatic volume or the grade of obstruction is weak
- Symptom quantification with the International Prostate Symptom Score (IPSS) helps to determine the severity of the disease, detects symptom progression and documents response to therapy
- With the IPSS the impact of urinary symptoms on quality of life can also be evaluated.

A certain proportion of aging men develop BPH usually combined with prostate enlargement. Of those, some but not all will suffer under LUTS. On the other hand some may have LUTS for reasons other than BPH (e.g. urethral stricture, stones, inflammation). Thus, the complex of symptoms now commonly referred to as LUTS is not specific for BPH. Lower urinary tract pathologies in aging men produce similar, if not identical, symptoms. Therefore, in patients with LUTS it is to establish that the symptoms are a result of BPH. Causes of symptoms not due to BPH can be excluded in a significant majority of patients by history, physical examination, and urinalysis. A medical history should be taken to identify other causes of voiding dysfunction. It should include questions for nocturia, weak stream, hesitancy, dribbling, gross hematuria and urinary tract infection.

- The symptoms of BPH include a wide spectrum of obstructive and irritative forms, which can appear in different severity. The symptoms represent the phases of urinary storing (irritative) and voiding (obstructive). Obstructive symptoms occur more frequently than irritative symptoms (see Chapter 3).

The obstructive symptoms can be explained by an elevated outflow resistance index of the prostatic urethra, the irritative symptoms may be explained by a secondary injury of the detrusor combined with a reduced compliance and detrusor instability. Both symptom groups are not specific for BPH, one can find them also in other diseases of the lower urinary tract (traumatic, inflammatory, postoperative) and in neurologic disorders (Table 10.1). At the beginning of the diagnostic process diseases like heart insufficiency or diabetes mellitus, which can produce nocturia and frequency as well, should be separated.

With progression of the disease some late symptoms or secondary diseases may occur like urinary tract infection, urinary incontinence, bladder calculi, urinary retention with hydronephrosis or renal insufficiency. The risk for acute urinary retention increases with age and baseline symptom severity. Additionally to the already specified symptoms some patients suffer from hematuria due to bladder neck varicosis.

BPH can be asymptomatic for a long time, yet it may lead to heavy complications like injury to the upper urinary tract or uremia. However, in most cases there are disturbing symptoms.

The natural course of disease in BPH is signed by phases of strongly marked symptoms alternating with asymptomatic intervals.

A single determination of symptoms will not be able to classify the prognostic outcome for a patient sufficiently. More important than the absolute value of a symptom score is the dynamic proceeding of symptom changes, which can be different depending on age.

Table 10.1 Differential diagnosis of BPH

Urological	Others
Prostate cancer	Neurologic bladder
Prostatitis	disorders
Bladder carcinoma	Right heart
Cystitis	insufficiency
Bladder calculi	Diabetes mellitus
Bladder neck sclerosis	Diabetes insipidus
Urethral stricture	Pelvic tumors
Urethral diverticulum	
Urethral calculi	
Urethral cancer	
Urethritis	

There is only a small relation between the prostate volume, the grade of obstruction and the extent of symptoms. Neither symptoms nor flow rate nor prostate volume measures can predict presence and degree of obstruction reliably. However, in most cases the symptoms decide for indication, kind and extension of therapy.

10.1 Which questionnaires and why?

In addition to the mere enumeration of symptoms by frequency of occurrence, the bother associated with the symptoms, interference with activities of daily living, and the impact the symptoms have on quality of life are important distinguishing characteristics.

Symptom quantification is important to determine the severity of the disease, to determine the progression of the disease over time, to identify the moment of necessary intervention, and to document the response to therapy.

For a quantitative measurement of symptoms patient voiding diaries, where the frequency of micturition and urine volume is recorded, may be helpful. However, the best instrument to assess the severity of symptoms in the initial evaluation or in monitoring the change in symptoms over timeis a validated symptom score.

A lot of scores exist which can measure symptom severity and quality of life. Scores in current use are stable over time and are able to reflect clinically important changes.

The International Prostate Symptom Score (IPSS) is now international standard. The IPSS was developed by the Measurement Committee of the American Urological Association (AUA) and is derived from the AUA 7 score described by Barry and colleagues. Extended by one question to quality of life the AUA Symptom Index has been accepted as IPSS by the WHO in 1991.

The IPSS represents a standardized symptom severity and frequency questionnaire. 7 questions are used, where each question can yield 0 to 5 points, producing a total symptom score from S0 to S35. Patients scoring 0 to 7 points are classified as mildly symptomatic, those scoring from 8 to 19 points as moderately symptomatic, and those scoring 20 to 35 points as severely symptomatic (see Chapter 3). This index score has been shown tobe an accurate reflection of a man's overall symptoms over the preceding month. Moreover, it has been determined that the annual change in symptoms is about 0.3 points per year.

- The IPSS should be used as the symptom-scoring instrument in the initial assessment of each patient presenting with LUTS.

It has been shown to be superior to an unstructured interview in quantifying symptom frequency and severity. The symptom score should also be the primary determinant of treatment response or disease progression in the follow-up period.

10.2 Can symptom severity alone be used to allocate treatment?

Most reports agree that the symptom score as decision tool for treatment may only be used in patients with mild symptoms, which can most appropriately be managed by a watchful waiting approach. Moreover, it is postulated that patients with moderate or severe symptoms might benefit from pharmacotherapy or prostatectomy. However, the score is not able to decide, which form of therapy might be the best for the individual case.

10.3 Can the symptom score be used as an outcome predictor?

The score seems to be a useful instrument in patients with moderate or severe symptoms. As men with mild symptoms have little room for improvement they do not experience high levels of symptom reduction following surgery.

- Other validated assessments are the International Continence Society male questionnaire and the Danish Prostatic Symptom Score (DAN-PSS), measuring symptom severity and frequency, the BPH Impact Index, measuring the impact of symptoms on activities of daily living.

In spite of the high value of these scores one has to consider some limitations:

1. The IPSS appears less reliable in men over 65 years old. A clear trend toward an increase in symptom scores with advancing age is noticeable in all reported studies.
2. Men report nocturia with accuracy but tend to overstate daytime frequency.
3. Correlation of the score to intermittency or the strength of stream seems to be poor.
4. Age and cultural factors may influence the validation of the score.

- Also, some patients may require an explanation of the questions to adequately understand their intent. The education level significantly affects the understanding of the symptom score. Patients with low education misrepresent their scores more often and to a higher degree, possibly predisposing them to inappropriate care.

- Careful linguistic validation needs to be undertaken prior to its use in non-English speaking nations. There is no question that differences in comprehension of the translated questionnaire as well as different perception of the symptoms are the cause for cross-cultural differences in symptom severity reported in the literature.
- There are numerous reports of symptom severity as expressed by IPSS correlating poorly with peak urinary flow rate, postvoid residual urine, prostatic size or pressure-flow study results. This lack of correlation has led to some questions raised about the validity of the IPSS. Similar insufficient correlations have been seen in many other diseases: Peak respiratory flow correlates poorly with patient's reports of the severity of their asthma. An explanation for this lack of correlation may be that the IPSS and physiological assessments measure different things.

To conclude: Several instruments were developed and validated to assess bother, interference, and disease-specific quality of life and sexual function. These instruments have not been as widely applied as the IPSS score. The IPSS is both valid and reliable in identifying the need to treat patients with BPH and in monitoring their response to therapy.

However, the IPSS cannot be used to establish the diagnosis of BPH. Men with a variety of lower urinary tract disorders (e.g. infection, tumor, neurogenic bladder disease) will have a high IPSS.

> The IPSS is the ideal instrument to grade symptom severity, to predict and monitor the response to therapy, and to detect symptom progression. However, although validated for its reliability and internal consistency it is not a replacement for personal discussion of symptoms with the patient.

A symptom score alone does not represent the morbidity as perceived by the individual patient. An intervention may make more sense for a moderately symptomatic patient who finds his symptoms very bothersome than for a severely symptomatic patient who finds his symptoms tolerable.

10.4 **Quality of life assessment**

The impact of urinary symptoms due th BPH on the quality of life is evaluated by question 8 of the IPSS. This question can yield 0 to 6 points, producing a total symptom score from L0 to L6.

However, this question measures the extent to which patients tolerate their symptoms rather than evaluating their quality of life. If one looks for a more specific instrument representing patients quality of life one should use the 36-item short-form health survey (SF36). This questionnaire is used to measure general health status and quality of life. Using this score, it has been shown that increasing symptom severity was associated with worsening physical condition, social functioning, vitality, mental health and perception of general health.

Other validated assessment instruments may be administered. Examples of these instruments are the International Continence Society male questionnaire, the BPH impact index which measures the impact of symptoms on activities of daily living and sexual function questionnaires.

References

Barry MJ, Fowler FJ, O'Leary MP, Holtgrewe HL, Mebust WK, Cockett ATK (1992) The American Urological Association symptom index for BPH *J Urol* **148**: 1549–57.

de la Rosette JJ, Witjes WP, Schäfer W, Abrams P, Donovan JL, Peters TJ, Millard RJ, Frimodt-Møller C, Kalomiris P (1998) Relationships between lower urinary tract symptoms and bladder outlet obstruction: results from the ICS-"BPH" study *Neurourol Urodyn* **17**: 99–108.

Johnson TV, Schoenberg ED, Abbasi A, Ehrlich SS, Kleris R, Owen-Smith A, Gunderson K, Master VA (2009) Assessment of the performance of the American Urological Association symptom score in 2 distinct patient populations *J Urol* **181**: 230–7.

Chapter 11

Diagnosis and assessment of BPH: objective parameters

Matthias Oelke

> ## Key points
>
> - There is no clear relationship between BPE, BPO, and LUTS; therefore, each component of the BPH-disease has to be separately evaluated and quantified
> - The diagnostic workup has to exclude other causes of prostatic enlargement, bladder outlet obstruction, and LUTS
> - BPH-associated complications should be detected at baseline
> - Assessment of BPH includes recommended and optional tests. After baseline investigation, the physician should be able to determine if and how the patient should be treated.

The terminus benign prostatic hyperplasia (BPH) describes the microscopic changes of the prostate which are characterized by benign growth of epithelial, muscular and/or fibrotic cells in the prostatic gland. Direct proof of microscopic BPH by prostate biopsies is not necessary during routine assessment and restricted to those men in whom discrimination between BPH, prostate carcinoma, and prostatitis is indicated.

BPH might cause benign prostatic enlargement (BPE), lower urinary tract symptoms (LUTS), or benign prostatic obstruction (BPO). However, not all men with BPH develop BPE, LUTS, or BPO and the development of one component is not necessarily associated with the development of other components (see Fig. 2.1).

> The diagnostic-workup has to exclude other causes of prostatic enlargement, bladder outlet obstruction, and LUTS.

11.1 Diagnostic strategy

The aim of the diagnostic work-up is to exclude other causes of prostatic enlargement, LUTS, or bladder outlet obstruction than BPH. A set of tests are used accordingly but these tests also provide information about the presence and severity of the three BPH-components. For diagnostic and differential diagnostic evaluation the following tests should be used in a risk adapted fashion (Table 11.1).

Once other causes of BPH have been excluded and each BPH-component has been quantified, the physician should also evaluate whether BPH-associated complications have already occurred (Table 11.2). Complications are directly or indirectly related to BPO and exclude conservative treatment.

Table 11.1 Tests for assessment and differential diagnosis of clinical BPH (LUTS, BPE, BPO)

RECOMMENDED (in all patients)	OPTIONAL (indicated in selected patients with BPH-disease)	NOT RECOMMENDED (but may be indicated in selected patients for further assessment of abnormalities)
• History • Physical examination (incl. DRE) • Questionnaire (e.g., IPSS) • Urine analysis (midstream) • Blood analysis (PSA, creatinine) • Uroflowmetry • Ultrasound (kidney, bladder-postvoid residual urine)	• Voiding chart • Urodynamic investigation	• Endoscopy (urethro-cystoscopy) • X-ray investigations (urethrography, cystography, voiding cystography, intravenous pyelography, CT) • MRI

Table 11.2 BPH-associated complications and tests for their assessment

BPH-associated complications	Test
Urinary tract infections	History, urine analysis (dipstick)
Haematuria	History, urine analysis (dipstick)
Postvoid residual urine	(Ultrasound) measurement of postvoid residual urine
Urinary retention	(Ultrasound) measurement of postvoid residual urine (>300 ml)
Bladder stones	Bladder ultrasound
Bladder diverticula	Bladder ultrasound
Bilateral hydronephrosis	Renal ultrasound
Renal insufficiency due to BPO	Measurement of serum-creatinine concentration, creatinine clearance

11.2 Digito-rectal examination (DRE)

Transanal palpation of the prostate with the physician's finger tip is used to judge

- Prostate size for evaluation of BPE
- Consistency of prostate parenchyma for screening of prostate carcinoma
- Pain of the gland for exclusion of prostatitis or prostate abscess
- Anal sphincter tone
- Rectum surface for exclusion of rectum carcinoma.

Prostate volume tends to be underestimated with DRE and is as high as 25% in glands >50 ml.

- The chance of detecting prostate cancer in patients with "BPH-LUTS" varies between 5–15%. Palpable tumours can be confirmed by a second investigator in 90%. However, DRE has a low sensitivity and specificity (approx. 33 and 50%, respectively) for detecting cancer.

11.3 International Prostate Symptom Score (IPSS)

Questionnaires are used to qualify and quantify LUTS. Questionnaires should be used in all patients at baseline and are able to objectively quantify treatment effects. IPSS questionnaire was validated and results are reliable, consistent, and stable. However, IPSS is not disease-, age-, or gender-specific and, therefore, can be used to evaluate LUTS in all patients independent of the underlying disease. Other questionnaires might be used instead if those had been validated (e.g., ICSmale, Madson-Iverson Score, or Dan-PSS).

11.3.1 The IPSS-questionnaire

- has 7 questions for symptom and 1 question for "quality of life" assessment
- symptom questions can be divided into bladder filling symptoms (irritative; IPSS questions 2, 4, and 7) and voiding symptoms (obstructive; IPSS questions 1, 3, 5, and 6)
- for each symptom question the patient can choose between 6 (0–5) different answers and indicate how frequently the symptom has appeared on average during a 24-hour period during the last 4 weeks
- total symptom score ranges between 0 and 35, thereby documenting a span between no symptoms (0) to maximum amount of symptoms (35)
- symptom scores between 0-7 indicate mild, 8-19 moderate, and 20–35 severe symptom severity. Medical or surgical treatment should be considered in men with symptom scores >7
- the eighth IPSS question evaluates how the patient would feel if bladder symptoms would remain for the rest of his life; the patient has seven answers to express symptom bother (0-6), thereby documenting a span between excellent (0) and very poor quality of life (6)
- bladder filling symptoms are associated with greater symptom bother than voiding symptoms
- greater symptom bother (4–6) implies need for treatment
- decrease ≥3 IPSS (questions 1-7) during treatment can be realized by the patient as symptom relief and is usually associated with decrease of symptom bother (question 8).

11.4 **Voiding chart**

Voiding charts are helpful to qualify and quantify LUTS. Voiding charts should be used in men who need further objective assessment of frequency and voided volume at baseline or during treatment.

- The patient is asked to document each void with time and volume over a continuous period of 24–48 hours to objectively assess voiding frequency during day and night as well as voided volumes (frequency-volume chart)
- Voiding charts are useful to discriminate between pollakisuria/nocturia due to bladder dysfunction, nocturnal polyuria, or increased fluid intake
- Nocturnal polyuria is defined as excretion ≥⅓ of the total daily urine volume during night (sleeping) period and is suspicious of increased fluid intake before sleeping, cardiac insufficiency, or insufficient vasopressin secretion
- It might also be useful in selected patients to document the amount of fluid intake, the severity of urgency, and the time of urinary incontinence.

11.5 **Urine analysis**

Dipstick or microscopic sediment analyses of mid-stream urine can detect leukocytes, nitrite, erythrocytes/haemoglobin, and glucose.

- **Leukocytes (leukocyte esterase activity)** are a sign of urinary tract infections which are usually caused by bacteria and might even be the only cause of LUTS. In approx. 90–95% of cases one of the following bacterial species causes urinary tract infections, of which *Escherichia coli* is responsible for the majority of infections (Table 11.3)
- In cases of leukocytes or positive leukocyte esterase activity, a urine sample should be send to microbiology lab where urine is cultured and the type and amount of bacteria as well as potential anti-bacterial drugs are identified. All urinary tract infections in elderly men are regarded as complicated and, therefore, the underlying causes should always be evaluated. Urinary tract infections with kidney involvement are the most frequent causes of renal insufficiency. Although approx. 20% of men with BPH develop urinary tract infections there is no relationship to postvoid residual urine
- **Nitrite:** Nitrate in the urine can be reduced to nitrite by the following bacteria of Table 11.3: *Escherichia coli*, *Proteus*, *Klebsiella*, *Pseudomonas*, and *Staphylococcus* species.

Table 11.3 Bacteria most frequently causing urinary tract infections in the community and hospitals (percentages may deviate in different regions and countries; adapted from Graham & Galloway 2001)

Bacteria	Community (%)	Hospital (%)
Escherichia coli[*]	69.4	50.8
Proteus mirabilis[*]	4.3	5.1
Klebsiella/Enterobacter species[*]	4.7	7.3
Enterococcus species[†]	5.5	11.9
Staphylococcus species[†]	4.0	8.4
Pseudomonas aeruginosa[*]	0	11.1
Others	12.1	5.4

[*] Gram negative, [†] Gram positive

- **Erythrocytes/haemoglobin:** Haematuria appears after rupture of superficial prostatic vessels in patients with BPE but also in patients with transitional cell carcinoma, stones, urinary tract infections, or glomerulonephritis. Bladder cancer, bladder stones, distal ureter stones, or urinary tract infections might even be the only cause of LUTS. All men with haematuria should be further assessed by ultrasound, urethro-cystoscopy, urine cytology, and X-ray investigations to exclude transitional cell carcinoma
- **Glucose:** Most urine dipsticks are also able to detect glucose which, in some men, is the first sign of diabetes or diabetes-associated bladder dysfunction (decreased bladder sensation, detrusor underactivity).

11.6 **Blood analysis**

Only determination of the serum concentrations of prostate-specific antigen (PSA) or creatinine is useful in patients with BPH-LUTS.

11.6.1 **Prostatic specific antigen (PSA)**

- PSA is a glycoproteine (molecular weight 33,000 Dalton; 237 aminoacids), produced by prostatic stromal cells, and is prostate- but not disease-specific. Total serum PSA concentration might be increased or decreased in certain patient groups (Table 11.4)
- For adequate judgment of serum PSA concentration, patient history and timing of PSA assessment is crucial

- Serum half-life is 3 days which has to be taken into account before analysis and for interpretation
- PSA can be used as a proxy parameter for prostate size

> 1 gram of BPH tissue increases serum PSA concentration by 0.3 ng/ml (in contrast to 1 gram of prostate cancer tissue that increases PSA concentration by 3.5 ng/ml on average).

- During treatment with 5α-reductase inhibitors (after 6-12 months of treatment with dutasteride or finasteride), PSA has to be doubled for correct judgement
- PSA screening for prostate cancer in the general population remains controversial but seems to be useful in elderly men with LUTS. The higher the PSA concentration the higher the chance of prostate cancer (Table 11.5). Prostate biopsies may be indicated in men with PSA-concentrations >4.0 ng/ml (or in those with palpable or visible tumours during DRE or prostate ultrasound, respectively)
- PSA-density (serum PSA concentration [ng/ml] divided by prostate volume [ml]; normal <0.15) in men with PSA concentrations 4-10 ng/ml, PSA-velocity (increase of serum PSA concentration over time; normal <0.75 ng/ml/year), and the proportion of free to total serum PSA concentration (normal >0.20) helps distinguishing between BPH and prostate cancer
- In men without prostate cancer, a higher serum PSA concentration is associated with BPH-disease progression (>1.6 ng/ml) and treatment benefit during 5α-reductase inhibitor therapy

Table 11.4 Causes for increased or decreased serum PSA concentrations	
PSA increased	**PSA decreased**
Benign prostatic enlargement (BPE)	After prostate tissue removal (e.g., TURP)
Prostatitis	After castration
Prostate carcinoma	Hypopituitarism
Prostate infarction	Androgen receptor defects (inherited)
After ejaculation	5α-reductase insufficiency (inherited)
Immediately after prostate manipulation: - digito-rectal examination - prostate biopsies - prostate operations	During treatment with: - 5α-reductase inhibitors - anti-androgens - LH-RH

Table 11.5 Risk of prostate cancer in patients with "normal" PSA concentration (≤4 ng/ml; adapted from Thompsen et al., 2004)

PSA concentration (ng/ml)	Risk of prostate cancer (%)
≤0.5	6.6
0.6 – 1.0	10.1
1.1 – 2.0	17.0
2.1 – 3.0	23.9
3.1 – 4.0	26.9

- lower PSA concentration (<1.3 ng/ml) is associated with higher treatment success during treatment with anti-muscarinic drugs.

11.6.2 Serum-creatinine

Serum-creatinine is used to judge renal function. However, increased serum concentration is only seen if ≥50% of nephrons are damaged. For better judgment of renal function, calculation of creatinine clearance is recommended (Cockroft-Gault formula):

$$\frac{(140 - age\ [years]) \times body\ weight\ [kg]}{(72 \times serum\text{-}creatinine\ [mg/dl])}$$

Serum-creatinine concentration or clearance is useful before administration of intravenous contrast media, which might cause acute renal failure in patients with renal insufficiency (creatinine concentration >180 μmol/l), and for adjustment of drug doses.

11.7 Uroflowmetry

- Measurement of urinary flow rate is a screening test to evaluate and quantify voiding at baseline and during follow-up. The following facts are important for correct judgment of uroflowmetry:
- the flow curve is a product of detrusor contraction strength and bladder outlet resistance
- in patients with abnormal voiding, uroflowmetry cannot distinguish between reduced contraction strength and increased bladder outlet resistance
- voided volume should exceed 150 ml
- maximum urinary flow rate (Q_{max}) and the shape of the flow curve are the most important parameters
- validation of flow parameters is always necessary and artefact correction may be required (Figure 11.1)

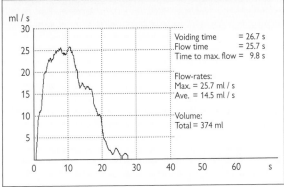

Fig 11.1 Flow curve of a patient with BPH and artefact pretending normal maximum urinary flow rate (Q_{max} >15 ml/s). Visual validation of flow parameters is required in each flow curve and manual correction of flow parameters might be necessary.

- Q_{max} is dependent on bladder volume: increasing Q_{max} between 150–500 ml but decreasing Q_{max} at higher volumes. Flow nomograms (e.g., Siroky nomogram) might be used to adequately judge Q_{max}
- uroflowmetry should be repeated if Q_{max} <15 ml/s
- Q_{max} ≥15 ml/s and a bell-shaped curve indicate normal voiding (Figure 11.2A). These men are unlikely to benefit from removal of prostatic tissue/prostate surgery
- only a minority of men with Q_{max} ≥15 ml/s have BPO (high-flow obstruction)
- Q_{max} <15 ml/s may be caused by BPO, urethral strictures, detrusor underactivity (hypocontractility), or dysfunctional voiding. The shape of the flow curve may indicate the underlying disease (Figures 11.2B–D)
- Q_{max} <11 ml/s is associated with disease progression and those men are likely to profit from medical or surgical intervention.

Fig 11.2 Prototypes of flow curves. (A) Q_{max} >15 ml/s and a bell-shaped curve indicate normal voiding function.
(B) Q_{max} <15 ml/s and a flattened curve are suspicious of bladder outlet obstruction or detrusor underactivity.
(C) Q_{max} <15 ml/s and a plateau-like curve are suspicious of urethral strictures. (D) Staccato-like curves are caused by dysfunctional voiding (detrusor-sphincter-dysfunction) or straining.

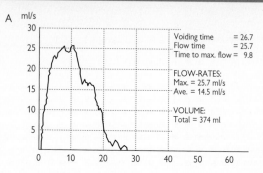

A

Voiding time   = 26.7
Flow time   = 25.7
Time to max. flow   = 9.8

FLOW-RATES:
Max. = 25.7 ml/s
Ave. = 14.5 ml/s

VOLUME:
Total = 374 ml

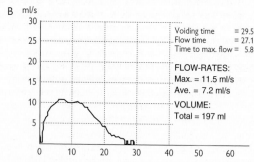

B

Voiding time   = 29.5
Flow time   = 27.1
Time to max. flow   = 5.8

FLOW-RATES:
Max. = 11.5 ml/s
Ave. = 7.2 ml/s

VOLUME:
Total = 197 ml

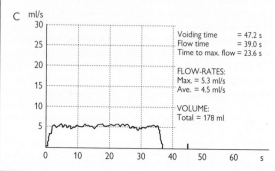

C

Voiding time   = 47.2 s
Flow time   = 39.0 s
Time to max. flow   = 23.6 s

FLOW-RATES:
Max. = 5.3 ml/s
Ave. = 4.5 ml/s

VOLUME:
Total = 178 ml

Fig 11.2 Continued

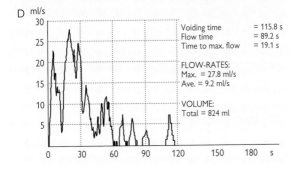

D ml/s

Voiding time = 115.8 s
Flow time = 89.2 s
Time to max. flow = 19.1 s

FLOW-RATES:
Max. = 27.8 ml/s
Ave. = 9.2 ml/s

VOLUME:
Total = 824 ml

11.8 Imaging

Imaging of the lower and upper urinary tract should preferably be done by ultrasound. However, intravenous pyelography or CT-scans might be indicated in those who have haematuria and are suspicious of having transitional cell carcinoma or upper urinary tract stones.

- **Renal ultrasound** aims to exclude upper urinary tract dilatation or renal pathologies (e.g., stones, renal cell cancer). Bilateral hydronephrosis indicates bladder dysfunction, whereas unilateral hydronephrosis is suspicious of retroperitoneal pathologies. Further assessment is necessary in all men with hydronephrosis. Measurement of renal parenchyma thickness can estimate renal function

- **Bladder ultrasound** by transabdominal positioning of the ultrasound probe aims to exclude bladder pathologies (e.g., stones, diverticula, tumours) and measure postvoid residual (PVR) urine. Assessment of bladder pathologies should be done with a full bladder and measurement of PVR immediately after voiding. The following facts about PVR are relevant for correct judgment:
  - all healthy men have PVR <12 ml
  - PVR >50 ml is considered pathological but a precise threshold value is not yet established
  - PVR measurement should be repeated in those with pathological values
  - urinary retention is defined as the inability to empty the bladder or PVR >300 ml
  - 25% of patients with BPO have PVR <50 ml and 30% without BPO have PVR >50 ml

- PVR as a single measure is unreliable for BPO assessment
- relevant PVR (>50 ml) is associated with a higher likelihood of disease progression; however, no threshold value has yet been established
- men with PVR >100 ml should receive active treatment
- **Prostate ultrasound** aims to determine the exact volume of the prostate by measuring the length, depth, and width of the gland. Transrectal ultrasound imaging of the prostate provides more reliable measures than transvesical imaging.

11.9 **Urodynamic evaluation**

Computer urodynamic investigation by simultaneous recording of bladder and abdominal pressures as well as urinary flow might be useful to evaluate the precise origin of LUTS, can discriminate between BPO and detrusor underactivity, and can quantify BPO. However, urodynamic evaluations are expensive, time-consuming and associated with morbidity; therefore, diagnostic profit has to be weighted against potential adverse events. Urodynamic evaluation is not necessary in the routine patient with BPH-LUTS but recommended before invasive treatment in men who:

- Cannot void ≥150 ml
- Have a maximum flow rate ≥15 ml/s
- Are <50 or >80 years of age
- Can void but have postvoid residual urine >300 ml
- Are suspicious of having neurogenic bladder dysfunction
- Have bilateral hydronephrosis
- Had radical pelvic surgery or
- Previous unsuccessful (invasive) treatment.

11.10 **Endoscopic evaluation**

Urethro-cystoscopy is not necessary in the routine patient with BPH-LUTS but might be useful to further assess haematuria and exclude lower urinary tract pathologies (e.g., transitional carcinoma, stones, or urethral strictures). The occlusion grade of prostatic urethra, distance between bladder neck and verumontanum, or the trabeculation grade of the bladder is not able to sufficiently diagnose BPO.

References

Barry MJ, Fowler FJ Jr, O'Leary MP, et al. (1992) The American Urological Association sympom index for benign prostatic hyperplasia. The Measurement Committee of the American Urological Association *J Urol* **148**: 1549–57.

Berges R, Dreikorn K, Höfner K, et al. (2009) Diagnostic and differential diagnostis of the benign prostatic syndrome (BPS): Guidelines of the German Urologists *Urologe* **48**: 1356–64.

Chancellor MB, Rivas DA, Keeley FX, et al. (1994) Similarity of the American Urological Association Symptom Index among men with benign prostatic hyperplasia (BPH), urethral obstruction not due to BPH and detrusor hyperreflexia without outlet obstruction *Br J Urol* **74**: 200–3.

El Din KE, de Wildt MJ, Rosier PF, et al. (1996) The correlation between urodynamic and cystoscopic findings in elderly men with voiding complaints *J Urol* **155**: 1018–22.

Graham JC, Galloway A (2001) The laboratory diagnosis of urinary tract infection. Best Practice No 167 *J Clin Pathol* **54**: 911–9.

Hald T (1989) Urodynamics in benign prostatic hyperplasia. A survey *Prostate*, Suppl 2: 69–77.

Homma Y, Gotoh M, Takei M, et al. (1998) Predictability of conventional tests for the assessment of bladder outflow obstruction in benign prostatic hyperplasia *Int J Urol* **5**: 61–6.

Kaplan SA (2004) AUA Guidelines and their impact on the management of BPH: An Update *Rev Urol* **6**(9): S46–52.

Leblanc G, Tessier J, Schick E (1995) The importance and significance of post-micturitional bladder residue in the evaluation of prostatism *Prog Urol* **5**: 511–4.

Madersbacher S, Alivizatos G, Nordling J, et al. (2004) EAU 2004 Guidelines on assessment, therapy and follow-up of elderly men with lower urinary tract symptoms suggestive of benign prostatic obstruction (BPH-Guidelines) *Eur Urol* **46**: 547–54.

Oelke M, Alivizatos G, Emberton M, et al. (2009) Guidelines on benign prostatic hyperplasia. In: *European Association of Urology pocket guidelines*. EAU guidelines office: 90–7.

Reynard JM, Yang Q, Donovan JL, et al. (1998) The ICS-"BPH" Study: uroflowmetry, lower urinary tract symptoms and bladder outlet obstruction *Br J Urol* **82**: 619–23.

Roehrborn CG, McConnell JD, Lieber MM, Waldstreicher J (1999) Serum prostate-specific antigen concentration is a powerful predictor of acute urinary retention and need for surgery in men with clinical benign prostatic hyperplasia. PLESS Study Group *Urology* **53**: 473–80.

Siroky MB, Olsson CA, Krane RJ (1980) The flow rate nomogram: II. Clinical correlations *J Urol* **123**: 208–10.

Thompson IM, Pauler DK, Goodman PJ, et al. (2004) Prevalence of prostate cancer among men with a prostate-specific antigen level ≤4.0 ng per milliliter *N Engl J Med* **350**: 2239–46.

Chapter 12

Watchful waiting and lifestyle issues associated with LUTS and BPH

Jørgen Nordling

> ### Key points
>
> - Watchful waiting combined with a teaching programme of self management is a highly viable option in men with not too bothersome LUTS
> - Malignancies in the lower urinary tract and complications to bladder outlet obstruction must be excluded before instituting such a programme.

Lower urinary tract symptoms (LUTS) are common in both males and females becoming increasingly more frequent with increasing age. Many males and females seek medical advice because of LUTS, but for many this is because of fear of an underlying severe disease. In males the fear of cancer and especially prostate cancer will often be the reason. The preliminary investigation of the patient will therefore focus primarily on diagnosing or excluding of cancer as the cause of LUTS.

Benign prostatic hyperplasia (BPH) is often the cause of LUTS in elderly males and often causes bladder outlet obstruction (BOO), so the exclusion of complications with BOO such as chronic urinary retention, deterioration of kidney function, etc. is another important issue in the preliminary evaluation of the male patient with LUTS. If cancer is excluded and no complications with BOO are found many feel relieved and in no need of further treatment and the patient and health practitioner might very well decide to do nothing for the time being.

This is traditionally called watchful waiting (WW) and it is customary in this sort of treatment to include education, reassurance, periodic monitoring and lifestyle interventions. Watchful waiting is a viable option for many men, but BPH is a progressive disease and a few complications with BOO or a larger number of worsening symptoms might occur over time making treatment necessary because of serious complications or desirable because of more troublesome symptoms.

12.1 Patient selection

- Male patient with mild to moderate LUTS
- Exclude cancer and complications with BOO
- Only slightly or moderately bothered by his symptoms.

This patient is suitable for a trial of watchful waiting. This will normally include advice on life style issues influencing LUTS including education, reassurance and to a certain degree future monitoring.

A large randomized, prospective study of 556 men comparing WW to transurethral resection of the prostate (TURP) with a 5 year follow up demonstrated only small differences in severe adverse events (Flanigan et al., 1998). Urinary retention was seen in 9 patients in the WW group compared to 1 in the TURP group (p=0,01) as the only significant severe adverse event being different between the groups.

After 5 years 36% of the patients randomized to WW had had a TURP and this group had the same trouble from LUTS as the group primarily randomized to TURP. It was however somewhat surprising that patients crossing over from WW to TURP had a slightly worse outcome in symptom resolution, peak flow rate and residual urine volume compared to those randomized to TURP. In this study 64% remained on WW at 5 years.

In a prospective study of 50 patients with mild LUTS only 2 (4%) had a TURP after 1 year (Netto et al., 1999), while in the above mentioned study of mild to moderate LUTS 65 (24%) underwent TURP within 3 years (Wasson et al., 1995) and 36% after 5 years (Flanigan et al., 1998). This is in accordance with the finding, that a lot of trouble was the only significant indicator of cross over from WW to TURP (Flanigan et al., 1998).

> The patient with LUTS and low trouble and no complications with BOO will be the patient most likely to be successful on a WW regime.

It has now been shown, that it is possible to decrease trouble from LUTS significantly by self management (Brown et al., 2007), thereby increasing the likelihood of a successful trial on WW.

12.2 Self management

Patients with bothersome LUTS will normally receive advice on life style and behavioural issues like fluid management, bladder re-training or re-scheduling of medicine. This has been termed self management (Richards, 1998).

Self management in the form of education, reassurance and periodic monitoring is however often performed in a very individual and different form. Christian T. Brown, Jan van der Meulen, Anthony R. Mundy, Elisabeth O'Flynn and Mark Emberton looked deeper into this using semi-structured interviews with health care professionals and a national UK practice survey (Brown et al., 2004). They found 57 items that were appropriate contained within:

12.3 Patient assessment prior to starting on a self-management programme

- Education and reassurance
  - Discuss the causes of LUTS, including normal prostate and bladder function
  - Discuss the natural history of BPH and LUTS, including the expected future symptoms
  - Reassure that no evidence of detectable prostate cancer has been found.
- Fluid management
  - Advise a daily fluid intake of 1500–2000 ml (minor adjustments for climate and activity), avoid inadequate or excessive intake on the basis of a frequency/volume chart
  - Advise fluid restriction when symptoms are most inconvenient, e.g. long journeys and when in public
  - Advise evening fluid restriction for nocturia (no fluid for 2 hours prior to retiring).
- Caffeine, alcohol
  - Avoid caffeine by substituting with alternatives, e.g. decaffeinated or non-caffeinated drinks
  - Avoid alcohol in the evening if nocturia is troublesome
  - Substitute large volume alcoholic drinks, e.g. a pint of beer with small volume alcoholic drinks, e.g. a short.
- Concurrent medication
  - Adjust the timing of medication with regard to the effect on the urinary system so as to improve LUTS at times of greatest inconvenience, e.g. long journeys and when out in public
  - Substitute anti hypertensive diuretics with suitable alternatives with less urinary effect (via the patient's GP).

- Types of toileting and bladder re-training
  - Advise men to double void
  - Advise urethral milking for men with post micturition dribble
  - Advise bladder retraining. Using distraction techniques (predetermined mind exercise, perineal pressure or pelvic floor exercises) aim to increase the minimum time between voids to 3 hours (daytime) and/or the minimum voided volume to between 200 and 400 ml (daytime). The urge to void should be suppressed for 1 min, then 5 mins, then 10 mins, etc. increasing on a weekly basis. Use frequency/volume charts to monitor progress.
- Avoid constipation—Implementation of a self managing program
  - Is done preferably by a specialist nurse or by a trained medical professional who has the time and expertise
  - Could be implemented by verbal or written means or by the help of a video
  - Assessment for compliance and symptom change initially every 4 weeks in the clinic or by telephone interview.

Follow up should include:
- Symptom assessment preferably using a validated score like the IPSS
- Quality of life/troublesome assessment preferably using a validated score.

Self management interventions should be delivered to men either on 1-to-1 or in small groups on no more than 10 persons.

In a prospective, randomized study self management it proved to be a very powerful tool (Brown et al., 2007). One hundred and forty men were randomized to either standard care or a self management regime.

Treatment failure was defined as an increase in IPSS of 3 or more, use of drugs to control LUTS, acute urinary retention or surgical intervention.

Treatment failure occurred in the first 6 months in more than half of the patients (61%) in the standard care group while treatment failures were much less and more evenly distributed in the self management group (Table 12.1).

Patients included in this study had from mild to severe symptoms and trouble and almost all had moderate symptoms. It therefore seems likely, that patients with moderate symptoms and trouble can be moved to the group with mild symptoms and trouble and therefore expect to have a greater possibility of a long-term trial of WW.

	Self management (N=73)	Standard care (N=67)	P value
Table 12.1 Outcome of self management versus standard care in a prospective, randomized study (Brown et al., 2007)			
3 month			
Treatment failure (%)	10	42	<0.0001
IPSS	10.7	16.4	<0.0001
BPH impact index	3.3	4.7	0.0003
AUA Qol score	2.8	3.4	<0.0001
6 month			
Treatment failure (%)	19	61	<0.0001
IPSS	10.4	16.9	<0.0001
BPH impact index	3.5	4.8	0.0008
AUA Qol score	2.6	3.3	0.0008
12 month			
Treatment failure	31	79	<0.0001
IPSS	10.2	15.4	<0.0001
BPH impact index	3.0	4.3	0.04
AUA Qol score	2.6	3.1	0.03

Watchful Waiting is a viable option in the handling of males with LUTS. Cancer, especially of the prostate, and complications with BOO must be excluded before starting the patient on WW. Patients with LUTS causing only mild trouble are most likely to have long-term success on WW. Patients with more troublesome LUTS can effectively decrease the troublesomeness of their LUTS by a self management programme.

References

Brown CT, van der Meulen J, Mundy AR, O'Flynn E, Emberton M (2004) Defining the components of a self-management programme for men with uncomplicated lower urinary tract symptoms: a consensus approach *Eur Urol* **46**(2): 254–62.

Brown CT, Yap T, Cromwell DA, Rixon L, Steed L, Mulligan K, et al. (2007) Self management for men with lower urinary tract symptoms: randomised controlled trial *BMJ* **334**(7583): 25.

Flanigan RC, Reda DJ, Wasson JH, Anderson RJ, Abdellatif M, Bruskewitz RC (1998) 5-year outcome of surgical resection and watchful waiting for men with moderately symptomatic benign prostatic hyperplasia: a Department of Veterans Affairs cooperative study *J Urol* **160**(1): 12–6.

Netto NR, Jr., de Lima ML, Netto MR, D'Ancona CA (1999) Evaluation of patients with bladder outlet obstruction and mild international prostate symptom score followed up by watchful waiting *Urology* **53**(2): 314–6.

Richards T (1998) Partnership with patients *BMJ* **316**(7125): 85–6.

Wasson JH, Reda DJ, Bruskewitz RC, Elinson J, Keller AM, Henderson WG (1995) A comparison of transurethral surgery with watchful waiting for moderate symptoms of benign prostatic hyperplasia. The Veterans Affairs Cooperative Study Group on Transurethral Resection of the Prostate *N Engl J Med* **332**(2): 75–9.

Chapter 13

Medical treatment of LUTS and BPH

Martin C. Michel

> ## Key points
>
> - Several mono- and combination treatments are available for LUTS/BPH
> - The risk/benefit ratio for each treatment depends on the patient to be treated
> - α-blockers provide rapid and effective symptom relief but do not prevent long-term complications
> - 5α-reductase inhibitors provide effective symptom relief and prevent long-term complications but work slower and effects on symptoms are smaller than those of α-blockers in most patients.

Lower urinary tract symptoms (LUTS) suggestive of benign prostatic hyperplasia (BPH) are highly prevalent in the elderly male population. This high prevalence necessitates that a large fraction of men with bothersome LUTS/BPH will, at least primarily, receive medical treatment. This coincides with the preference of most patients. This chapter will review specific features of various types of available medical treatments and their combinations and discuss their rational differential use.

13.1 Phytotherapy

Extracts from several plants have been tested for the treatment of LUTS/BPH. Most of these studies have two general problems:

- Firstly, two extracts obtained from the same plant do not necessarily contain the same active ingredients, neither qualitatively or quantitatively, due to differences in plant sources, harvesting and extraction methods

- Secondly, most plant extract studies have included small patient numbers, short observation periods and/or outcome measures which are distinct from those used in most other studies.

Among all plant extracts, most studies have been performed with extracts of saw palmetto (*Serenoa repens*). According to the most recent meta-analysis by the Cochrane collaboration, extracts of this plant do not provide greater benefit than placebo (Tacklind et al., 2009). Some earlier studies may partly have been positive because of blinding problems as saw palmetto extracts have a distinct smell.

In conclusion, plant extracts cannot be recommended for routine treatment of LUTS/BPH patients due to insufficient data supporting their use.

13.2 α-Blockers

Based upon the role of $_1$-adrenoceptors, specifically $_{1A}$-adrenoceptors, in the contraction of prostate smooth muscle it has long been assumed that antagonists of these receptors (blockers, ARBs) improve LUTS/BPH primarily by relaxing smooth muscle and hence reducing bladder outlet obstruction. However, more recent data demonstrate that ARBs as a class have only little if any effect on obstruction and that improvements of obstruction in individual patients do not correlate with those on symptoms (Barendrecht et al., 2008). Thus, it remains to be determined how precisely α-adrenoceptor blockade leads to LUTS/BPH improvement. Nevertheless, two factors appear certain.

- Firstly, their beneficial effects involve predominantly if not exclusively the $_{1A}$-subtype as drugs selective for this subtype such as tamsulosin and, even more importantly, silodosin are similarly effective as those blocking all subtypes
- Secondly, ARBs act on symptoms only and do not lead to inhibit prostate growth despite earlier reports on possible effects on apoptosis by some representatives of this class (Kyprianou et al., 2009). Whether the clinical effects involve the spinal cord and/or the urinary bladder as sites of action remains to be determined.

> When used in adequate doses all ARBs are equally effective (Table 13.1).

The ARBs are the most effective form of medical treatment with regard to symptom reduction. Their beneficial effects occur independently of prostate size and have a rapid onset of action, i.e. within hours to days, except for drugs requiring dose-titration upon initiation of treatment for safety reasons. The symptom improvement is maintained over many years. However, after several years of treatment BPH consequences such as acute urinary retention may occur and/or patients may ultimately require surgical treatment.

Thus, in controlled studies (typically involving a single-blind placebo run-in period) the IPSS improves by about 35–40% whereas Q_{max} increases by about 20–25% (Djavan et al., 2004). In observational open-label studies representing real-life rather than clinical study settings, symptom improvements typically are greater reaching up to 50% for IPSS and up to 40% for Q_{max}.

Table 13.1 Formulations and standard doses of clinically available α_1-Adrenoceptor antagonists

Drug	Dose
α_1-Adrenoceptor antagonists	
Alfuzosin	
Immediate release	3 × 2.5 mg
Sustained release	2 × 5 mg
Extended release	1 × 10 mg
Doxazosin	
Immediate release	1 × 4–8 mg
Gastro-intestinal therapeutic system	1 × 4–8 mg
Silodosin	1 × 4–8 mg
Tamsulosin*	
Modified release	1 × 0.4 mg
Oral controlled absorption system	1 × 0.4 mg
Terazosin immediate release	1 × 5–10 mg

* In some Asian countries the registered tamsulosin dose is 0.2 mg/d, although there are no published data demonstrating that the dose-response relationship differs between Asians and other ethnicities; in the Americas 0.8 mg/d is also registered, which may be associated with minor increases in efficacy at the cost of a reduced tolerability. Adapted from Michel MC, de la Rosette JJMCH. Medical treatment of lower urinary tract symptoms suggestive of benign prostatic hyperplasia. *Eur Urol Suppl* 2009; **8**:496–503.

While ARBs generally are well tolerated, frequent side effects include asthenia, dizziness and (orthostatic) hypotension. Interestingly, these adverse events appear to occur less frequently with the $_{1A}$-selective tamsulosin and silodosin than with the non-subtype-selective doxazosin and terazosin. However, alfuzosin, which chemically and with regard to lack of subtype-selectivity is closer to doxazosin and terazosin than to tamsulosin, also has a low incidence of side effects.

Clinically, this becomes most important in subjects who already are prone to orthostatic hypotension due to concomitant disease or medication with other vasodilating drugs including phosphodiesterase (PDE) type 5 inhibitors used in the treatment of erectile dysfunction (Barendrecht et al., 2005). These findings suggest that pharmacokinetic factors such as selective partitioning into lower urinary tract tissues and/or overall smooth pharmacokinetics may be at least as important as subtype-selectivity for an overall good tolerability. Two specific side effects deserve special notice:

- *Firstly*, abnormal ejaculation, now recognized to represent (relative) anejaculation rather than retrograde ejaculation, apparently occurs more frequent with tamsulosin and even more so with silodosin as compared to other ARBs (van Dijk 2006). Thus, this adverse event apparently is linked to selectivity for α_{1A}-adrenoceptors; while this probably relates to effects on the vas deferens, it remains unclear why the non-subtype-selective drugs are less prone to this side effect as they also block the $_{1A}$-adrenoceptor in clinically used doses. Abnormal ejaculation occurs mostly in younger patients, and if it occurs may warrant the use of a drug where this occurs less frequently

- *Secondly*, it has been recognized that patients undergoing ARB treatment may exhibit an intra-operative floppy iris syndrome while undergoing cataract surgery. This may occur more frequently upon use of tamsulosin than with other agents from this class. However, in all cases these ocular effects have been manageable without lasting complications for the patient, e.g. by the use of intracameral application of a $_1$-adrenoceptor agonist such as phenylephrine.

In conclusion, ARBs are a suitable first-line option for the medical treatment of LUTS/BPH. All have a similar efficacy but they may differ in tolerability.

13.3 5α-reductase inhibitors

Two isoforms of 5α-reductase exist, type 1 and 2, of which finasteride inhibits only one whereas dutasteride inhibits both. However, the available clinical data do not support the notion that inhibition that inhibition of both isoforms is association with qualitatively or quantitatively different efficacy or tolerability.

Inhibition of 5α-reductase leads to a reduction in prostate size by about 20% (and of PSA by about 50%) which is believed to be the basis for the relief of LUTS by 5α-reductase inhibitors (ARIs) (Naslund et al., 2007).

In line with their mechanism of action, the beneficial effects of ARIs on LUTS develop during the course of several months. In studies with 6 months to 4 years of duration, symptom relief by ARIs in direct comparative studies was less than that by ARBs in non-selected populations (McConnell et al., 2003); however, in patients with large prostate it may be similar to or even larger than that of ARBs (Roehrborn et al., 2008). Symptom reduction by ARIs depends on prostate size, i.e. may be close to placebo effects with prostates of less than 40 ml (Boyle et al. 1996). Long-term, i.e. multi-year, ARI treatment reduces the risk of AUR or the risk of requiring surgical treatment (McConnell et al., 2003), and this may also be detectable with prostate size of <40 ml.

> In patients with large prostates the effect of 5α-reductase inhibitors it may be similar to or even larger than that of ARBs (Roehrborn et al., 2008).

While ARIs are generally well tolerated, their most frequent side effects relate to sexual function and include reduced libido, erectile dysfunction and, less frequently, abnormal ejaculation (Naslund et al., 2007).

In conclusion, ARIs are a suitable first-line option for the long-term medical treatment of LUTS/BPH in men with large prostate. No clinically relevant differences have been noted between the available agents.

Table 13.2 Formulations and standard doses of clinically available 5α-reductase inhibitors	
5α-reductase inhibitors	
	Dose
Dutasteride	1 × 0.5 mg
Finasteride	1 × 5 mg

13.4 Anticholinergics

Muscarinic receptor antagonists have long been considered potentially harmful in the treatment of LUTS/BPH. This was based upon the idea that they will cause bladder smooth muscle relaxation which, in combination with bladder outlet obstruction, may lead to urinary retention. On the other hand, it has been realized in recent years that many of the LUTS typically attributed to BPH in men also occur in women where they are attributed to an OAB. This has raised the question whether indeed all LUTS in men are caused by BPH and whether at least some of them may rather be explained by male OAB, possibly concomitant with BPH. Moreover, it has been realized that the human prostate expresses muscarinic receptors, actually at densities exceeding those of α_1-adrenoceptor expression (Witte et al., 2008).

Based on such ideas various studies have been performed in recent years to evaluate the safety and efficacy of muscarinic receptor antagonists in men with LUTS (Lee et al., 2008). Most of these studies have used propiverine or tolterodine as the muscarinic antagonists and been performed with these drugs as an add-on to ARB treatment and/or in men with an insufficient clinical response to ARBs.

While minor elevations of residual volume have been observed in some but not other studies, a surprising overall finding has been that no dramatic increases in urinary retention were observed. On the other hand, those studies consistently reported improved symptoms. Of note is one major study in which inclusion criteria and endpoints of both classical BPH and OAB studies were applied concomitantly (Kaplan et al., 2006). This study compared placebo, tamsulosin, tolterodine and the combination of the two active treatments during a 12 week observation period. Interestingly, in a study population defined that way, neither tamsulosin nor tolterodine alone exhibited the efficacy over placebo expected based on previous BPH or OAB studies, respectively. However, their combination was highly effective against most endpoints.

These studies suggest that muscarinic receptor antagonists not only cause little harm in men, even in the presence of BPH, and actually may be beneficial for their storage LUTS, particularly in combination with an ARB. However, several caveats apply before muscarinic receptor antagonists alone or in combination can be recommended for the routine treatment of male LUTS.

- Firstly, it remains to be clarified which men benefit from muscarinic receptor antagonists.
- Secondly, the place of such drugs in the therapeutic cascade of male LUTS remains to be determined.

Finally, although no major increases in acute urinary retention have been observed with muscarinic receptor antagonists in men, the currently available studies remain vastly underpowered to detect e.g. a doubling in retention rates, largely because acute urinary retention occurs so rarely (1-2 cases in 100 patient years of men with LUTS/BPH).

In conclusion, muscarinic receptor antagonists are a promising option for the treatment of male LUTS but the currently available data are insufficient for definitive treatment recommendations.

13.5 **PDE5-inhibitors**

PDE5 inhibitors were originally introduced for the treatment of erectile dysfunction. As this condition occurs frequently in men with

LUTS/BPH which in turn frequently receive ARB treatment, concerns have been raised whether the combination of PDE5 inhibitors and ARBs will be safe with regard to blood pressure effects[3]. Meanwhile it has become clear that such a combination is not necessarily dangerous, particularly when ARBs with limited cardiovascular effects such as alfuzosin, silodosin or tamsulosin are used.

> Concomitantly it has been realized that PDE5 inhibitors may cause smooth muscle relaxation not only in the penis but also in the bladder outflow tract.

This led to the proposal that such drugs may actually be beneficial in men with LUTS/BPH. Based upon this idea several controlled clinical studies with the PDE5 inhibitors sildenafil, tadalafil and vardenafil have been performed in LUTS/BPH patients (Anderson et al., 2007). In contrast to the studies in erectile dysfunction, which are largely based on on-demand administration of the drugs, those in LUTS/BPH were based on daily administration. They have consistently reported symptom improvement of a magnitude similar to that of ARBs, although little direct comparative data are available. On the other hand and in contrast to the original hypothesis, PDE5 inhibitors failed to increase Q_{max}.

While it has been argued that this may at least partly relate to study design, it indicates that LUTS improvement by PDE5 inhibitors apparently are not fully explained by smooth muscle relaxation but alternative hypotheses have not been proven. Meanwhile a low dose administration of tadalafil has been approved in many countries for daily use in erectile dysfunction, and this treatment scheme may also receive regulatory approval for LUTS/BPH in the future. However, at current prices of such drugs their use in LUTS/BPH may remain limited.

In conclusion, PDE5 inhibitors are effective in the treatment of LUTS/BPH but currently remain an expensive off-label option.

13.6 **Combination therapy**

Various combinations of the above-mentioned medication groups are possible and have been evaluated in controlled studies. Although combination treatment sometimes provides additional benefit over monotherapy, it is a general observation from all of these studies that combination treatment not only implies greater cost for medication but always comes with an increased risk for adverse events. Such elevated risk becomes particularly important when a combination treatment is planned for long-term (multi-year) treatment.

The overall benefit of combination treatment for an individual patient, therefore, needs to be evaluated against the background of the individual symptom severity and risk for complications of that patient as the balance between potentially greater efficacy and a higher risk for side effects.

The combination of ARB and ARI has been tested most frequently, and at least 6 studies between 6 months and more than 4 years of duration are now available. In studies up to two years, the combination of ARB and ARI did not reduce LUTS to a greater extent than the ARB alone. A benefit of an ARB/ARI combination over use of an ARB alone was found only in studies of more than two years of duration (McConnell et al., 2003). This combination was also superior over both ARB and ARI monotherapy with regard to reducing the risk for a clinically defined endpoint of disease progression after several years. Based upon these data an ARB/ARI combination appears only promising to use if indeed a long-term medical treatment is planned and has been discussed with the patient. Moreover, it should be noted that the risk of disease progression is mostly relevant for patients at high risk for progression. On the other hand, in such high risk patient a risk reduction of about 50% may be too little, and these patients may actually benefit more from surgical treatments, including minimally invasive ones.

Another combination is between ARBs and muscarinic receptor antagonists. Actually, most studies on the use of muscarinic receptor antagonists in men with LUTS have been performed as add-on to existing ARB treatment. While this combination appears attractive, particularly for the bothersome storage symptoms, it remains to be determined which patients are suitable for such a combination as compared to those most likely to benefit from ARB or muscarinic receptor antagonist treatment alone.

The combination of ARBs and PDE5 inhibitors has been evaluated at least in pilot studies with very promising results with regard to additive efficacy (Kaplan et al., 2007). However, these findings need to be confirmed in larger controlled studies. Moreover, this combination at present appears to be the most expensive option for medical treatment of LUTS/BPH and only appears safe when ARBs with minimal cardiovascular effects are chosen.

Other combinations are also possible including triple medications, but it always needs to be kept in mind that any additional drug increases the risk for adverse events. Hence, any additional benefit must be weighed against such increased risk. One combination which appears very attractive on theoretical grounds but has not yet been studied systematically is that between an ARI and a PDE5 inhibitor.

Many options exist for the medical treatment of LUTS/BPH. The two classical options, ARBs and ARIs, as well as their combination have clearly defined clinical risk/benefit profiles. Muscarinic receptor antagonists and PDE5 inhibitors have shown promising findings in multiple studies but the place of these agents for routine use remains to be defined. This is particularly true for combination of these drugs with ARBs or ARIs.

Acknowledgements: Within this therapeutic area, the author has received research funding, lecturer and/or consultant honoraria from Astellas, Boehringer Ingelheim, Eli Lilly, Pfizer, Recordati and Schwarz Pharma.

References

Andersson K-E, Ückert S, Stief C et al. Phosphodiesterases (PDEs) and PDE inhibitors for treatment of LUTS. *Neurourol Urodyn* 2007; **26**: 928–933.

Barendrecht MM, Abrams P, Schumacher H et al. Do α_1-adrenoceptor antagonists improve lower urinary tract symptoms by reducing bladder outlet resistance? *Neurourol Urodyn* 2008; **27**: 226–230.

Barendrecht MM, Koopmans RP, de la Rosette JJMCH et al. Treatment for lower urinary tract symptoms suggestive of benign prostatic hyperplasia: the cardiovascular system. *BJU Int* 2005; **95** Suppl. 4: 19–28.

Boyle P, Gould AL, Roehrborn CG. Prostate volume predicts outcome of treatment of benign prostatic hyperplasia with finasteride: meta-analysis of randomized clinical trials. *Urology* 1996; **48**: 398–405.

Djavan B, Chapple C, Milani S et al. State of the art on the efficacy and tolerability of alpha1-adrenoceptor antagonists in patients with lower urinary tract symptoms suggestive of benign prostatic hyperplasia. *Urology* 2004; **64**: 1081–1088.

Kaplan SA, Gonzalez RR, Te AE. Combination of alfuzosin and sildenafil is superior to monotherapy in treating lower urinary tract symptoms and erectile function. *Eur Urol* 2007; **51**: 1717–1723.

Kaplan SA, Roehrborn CG, Rovner ES et al. Tolterodine and tamsulosin for treatment of men with lower urinary tract symptoms and overactive bladder. A randomized controlled trial. *J Am Med Assoc* 2006; **296**: 2319–2328.

Kyprianou N, Vaughan TB, Michel MC. Apoptosis induction by doxazosin and other quinazoline α_1-adrenoceptor antagonists: a new mechanism for cancer treatment? *Naunyn-Schmiedeberg's Arch Pharmacol* 2009; **380**: 473–477.

Lee K-S, Lee HW, Han DH. Does anticholinergic medication have a role in treating men with overactive bladder and benign prostatic hyperplasia? *Naunyn-Schmiedeberg's Arch Pharmacol* 2008; **377**: 491–501.

McConnell JD, Roehrborn CG, Bautista O et al. The long-term effect of doxazosin, finasteride, and combination therapy on the clinical progression of benign prostatic hyperplasia. *New Engl J Med* 2003; **349**: 2387–2398.

Michel MC, de la Rosette JJMCH. Medical treatment of lower urinary tract symptoms suggestive of benign prostatic hyperplasia. *Eur Urol Suppl* 2009; **8**: 496–503.

Naslund MJ, Miner M. A review of the clinical efficacy and safety of 5α-reductase inhibitors for the enlarged prostate. *Clin Ther* 2007; **29**: 17–25.

Roehrborn CG, Siami P, Barkin J et al. The effects of dutasteride, tamsulosin and combination therapy on lower urinary tract symptoms in men with benign prostatic hyperplasia and prostatic enlargement: 2-year results from the ComAT study. *J Urol* 2008; **179**: 616–621.

Tacklind J, MacDonald R, Rutks I et al. Serenoa repens for benign prostatic hyperplasia. *Cochrane Database Syst Rev* 2009.

van Dijk MM, de la Rosette JJMCH, Michel MC. Effects of α1-adrenoceptor antagonists on male sexual function. *Drugs* 2006; **66**: 287–301.

Witte LPW, Chapple CR, de la Rosette JJMCH et al. Cholinergic innervation and muscarinic receptors in the human prostate. *Eur Urol* 2008; **54**: 326–334.

Chapter 14

Interventional treatment: open prostatectomy

C. Gratzke and Christian G. Stief

> ### Key points
>
> - Open prostatectomy results in excellent functional results, associated with a low morbidity and mortality rate
> - Because it's easy to perform the technique, and because of its low technical demands, it represents the standard technique for patients with lower urinary tract symptoms due to significant benign prostate enlargement and bladder outlet obstruction in the majority of countries
> - Despite the promising results of minimally-invasive techniques such as laparoscopic and robotic prostate enucleation, these techniques are still confined to centres of excellence.

Open prostatectomy has been the primary treatment option for patients with lower urinary tract symptoms due to benign prostatic enlargement (BPE) and benign prostatic obstruction (BPO) for decades. Two main approaches for open prostatectomy emerged during the early part of the 20th century: the suprapubic transvesical and retropubic transcapsular routes (Freyer, 1912; Millen, 1947).

While open prostatectomy is invasive and requires a lower midline incision with subsequently relatively long hospitalization and convalescence time, it results in an excellent functional outcome and low reoperation rates (Tubaro et al., 2001; Varkarakis et al., 2004; Naspro et al., 2006; Gratzke et al., 2007). Advancements in laparoscopic urological expertise led to the development of laparoscopic as well as robotic simple prostatectomy (Mariano et al., 2002; Baumert et al., 2006; Mariano et al., 2006; Sotelo et al., 2008; McCullough et al., 2009). There is growing evidence that these minimally-invasive techniques are effective and safe options to open prostatectomy.

All techniques have to be compared to the gold standard in the surgical treatment of lower urinary tract symptoms, which is the minimal-invasive transurethral resection of the prostate (TURP).

14.1 Open prostatectomy

Indications for open prostatectomy include not only the treatment for adenomas greater than 80 to 100 cm (Naspro et al., 2006), but also and especially coexistent pathological conditions such as bladder diverticulum, bladder stones and inguinal hernia (Han et al., 2002). The first technqiue ever described was the perineal approach, more than 2000 years ago, which was performed until suprapubic transvesical prostatectomy was popularized by Freyer at the beginning of th 20th century (Freyer, 1912). In 1945, Millin published the retropubic transcapsular prostatectomy for the first time (Millen, 1947; Bruskewitz, 1999).

In most countries with fewer health care resources, lack of endoscopic equipment and endourological experience, open prostatectomy is the standard technique, which is confirmed today by incidence rates in developed countries between 13% to 40% of all cases (Bruskewitz, 1999; Seretta et al., 2002).

14.1.1 Functional outcome

There is abundant evidence that open prostatectomy results in excellent functional results with low morbidity and mortality. In a large prospective study including more than 900 patients, post-void residual volume as well as urinary flow rate had improved significantly at discharge (Gratzke et al., 2007) (Table 14.1.(Freyer, 1912)). Peak flow rate increased significantly from a baseline of 10.6 ± 6.4 ml/sec to 23.1 ± 10.5 ml/sec, while post-void residual urine decreased significantly from 145.1 ± 152.8 ml to 17.5 ± 34.8 ml at discharge. Mean operative time was 80.8 ± 34.2 minutes, while mean enucleated tissue was 84.8 ± 44 gm. Incidental carcinoma of the prostate was found on histological examination in 3.1% of this PSA-screened population. Similar outcomes for functional results at patients' discharge were reported by Adam et al. in a retrospective study (Adam et al., 2004). In as small prospective study, Tubaro et al. showed a decrase in symptoms as measured with the International Prostate Symptom Score (IPSS) from 19.9 ± 4.4 to 1.5 ± 2.7 and an increase in quality of life one year after surgery (QoL-score decreased from 4.9 ± 1 to 0.2 ± 0.4) (Tubaro et al., 2001). Maximum flow rate improved from

9.1 ± 5.3 to 29.0 ± 8.9 ml/sec, while residual urine decreased from 128 ± 113 to 8 ± 18 ml. These excellent functional results were shown to last up to 5 years, as shown in prospective and retrospective analyses (Varkaraksis et al., 2004; Naspro et al., 2006; Kuntz et al., 2008). At five years, the symptom index (AUA-SI) had dropped from 21.0 ± 3.6 to 3.0 ± 1.7, while peak urinary flow rates had increased from 3.6 ± 3.8 to 24.4 ± 7.4 ml/sec 16. Post-void residual volume had decreased from 292 ± 191 ml to 5.3 ± 11.2 ml.

Table 14.1

Authors	Year	Study design	Follow-up	N=Patients	Symptom score		QoL		Qmax		PVR	
					Pre-op	Post-op	Pre-op	Post-op	Pre-op	Post-op	Pre-op	Post-op
Adam et al[15]	2004	Retrospective	At discharge	201	-		-		6.46 ±6	22.05 ±10	170.97 ±258	7.0 ±2.3
Gratzke et al[1]	2007	Prospective	At discharge	868	IPSS	20.7 ±7.6	-	-	10.6 ±6.4	23.1 ±10.5	145.1 ±152.8	17.5 ±34.8
Tubaro et al[1]	2001	Prospective	12 months	32	IPSS	19.9 ±4.4	1.5 ±2.7	4.9 ±1.0	0.2 ±0.4	9.1 ±5.3	29.0 ±8.9	128 ±113	8±18
Naspro et al[2]	2006	Prospective	24 months	39	IPSS	21.6 ±3.24	8.1 ±7.1	4.44 ±0.96	1.66 ±0.76	8.32 ±2.37	20.11 ±5.8	-	-
Varkarakis et al[1]	2004	Retrospective	41.8.5.6 months	151	IPSS	24.9 ±4.8	1.6 ±0.9	4.7 ±0.6	0.5 ±0.7	7.2 ±1.8	23.7 ±3	116.9 ±42	11.94 ±6.5
Kuntz et al[16]	2008	Prospective	60 months	32	AUASS	21.0 ±3.6	3.0 ±1.7			3.6 ±3.8	24.4 ±7.4	292 ±191	5.3 ±11.2

Urodynamic changes post-operatively were also assessed over time 3. The authors showed an obstruction relief starting with a 3-month follow-up and reaching a plateau at 24 months (Schäfer grade/LinPURR 3.1 at baseline versus 0.8 12 months post surgery).

> Based on these data, it is valid to assume that open prostatectomy provides long-lasting functional improvements in association with an increase in quality of life.

14.1.2 Morbidity and mortality

The development of open prostatectomy has seen a steady decrease in morbidity and mortality. The main perioperative complications include urinary tract infections (UTI) (2.6–12.9 %), surgical revision due to severe bleeding (0–3.7%) and blood transfusions (0–24%) (Naspro et al., 2006; Gratzke et al., 2007; Kuntz et al., 2008). Mortality rates were described as low as 0–0.2%. Late complications included bladder neck contractions, urethral strictures needing surgical treatment (up to 6.7 %) and dysuria (up to 3.3%). Erectile function, which was measured with the erectile function domain of the IIEF, showed no significant reduction in the follow-up period from baseline in either group (Naspro et al., 2006).

14.2 **Minimally-invasive simple prostatectomy**

14.2.1 **Laparoscopic simple prostatectomy**

The feasibility of laparoscopic simple prostatectomy was first described in 2002 by Mariano et al. (Mariano et al., 2002). Four years later, the same group reported results from 60 patients who had undergone laparoscopic prostatectomy (Mariano et al., 2006). The average prostate weight was 144.50 +/− 41.74 gm, with mean operative time 138.48 +/− 23.38 minutes and estimated blood loss of 330.98 +/− 149.52 ml. No patient required transfusions or conversion to open surgery, and the complication rate post-operatively was low. The erectile function was preserved in all those patients who were potent before surgery. No urinary incontinence was reported by patients. As with most laparoscopic approaches, short hospital stay and early return to normal activity were considered to be the main advantages. To date, reports from several centres have confirmed technical feasibility and safety of laparoscopic simple prostatectomy (Nadler et al., 2004; van Velthoven et al., 2004; Baumert et al., 2006).

In a non-randomized, comparative study, 280 consecutive patients underwent prostatectomy either by the extraperitoneal laparoscopic transcapsular (Millin) or open transvesical (Freyer) approach. There was no significant difference in uroflow rate, mean IPSS, operative blood loss, total time of continuous bladder irrigation and complication rate between the groups. Mean operative time was significantly longer in the laparoscopy group, while hospital stay and length of catheterization was significantly shorter (McCullough et al., 2009).

14.2.2 **Robot-assisted simple prostatectomy**

The first reports about robot-assisted transperitoneal simple prostatectomies were published by Sotelo and co-workers in 2008 for 7 patients (Sotelo et al., 2008). Average operative time was 205 minutes, hospital stay 1.4 days and Foley catheter duration 7 days. No complications were documented. Considerable improvements from baseline were noted in IPSS (22 vs 7.25) and maximum urine flow (17.75 vs 55.5 ml/sec). Advocators of the robotic approach postulate advantages such as three-dimensional vision, six degrees of freedom in the instrument's movements, and downscaling of movements, which are believed to allow the surgeon greater precision and vision. While a number of feasibility studies have been reported (Yuh et al., 2008; Bucher et al., 2009), it will be interesting to see whether this technique will gain broad acceptance in the near future.

References

Adam C, Hofstetter A, Deubner J et al. (2004) Retropubic transvesical prostatectomy for significant prostatic enlargement must remain a standard part of urology training *Scand J Urol Nephrol* **38**: 472.

Baumert H, Ballaro A, Dugardin F et al. (2006) Laparoscopic versus open simple prostatectomy: a comparative study *J Urol* **175**: 1691.

Bruskewitz R (1999) Management of symptomatic BPH in the US: who is treated and how? *Eur Urol* **36**(3): 7.

Bucher, JH, Engel, N et al. (2009) Preperitoneal robotic prostate adenomectomy *Urology* **73**: 811.

Freyer P (1912) One thousand cases of total enuceation of the prostate for radical cure of enlargement of that organ *Br Med J* **868**.

Gratzke C, Schlenker B, Seitz M et al. (2007) Complications and early postoperative outcome after open prostatectomy in patients with benign prostatic enlargement: results of a prospective multicenter study *J Urol* **177**: 1419.

Han M, Alfert H, Partin A (2002) Retropubic and suprapubic open prostatectomy. In: *Campbell's Urology* Edited by PCR Walsh, Vaughan ED, Wein AJ. Philadelphia: Saunders., 8th edition., pp. 1423–1433.

Kuntz RM, Lehrich K, Ahyai SA (2008) Holmium laser enucleation of the prostate versus open prostatectomy for prostates greater than 100 grams: 5-year follow-up results of a randomised clinical trial *Eur Urol* **53**: 160.

Mariano M.B, Graziottin TM, Tefilli, MV (2002) Laparoscopic prostatectomy with vascular control for benign prostatic hyperplasia *J Urol* **167**: 2528.

Mariano MB, Tefilli MV, Graziottin TM et al. (2006) Laparoscopic prostatectomy for benign prostatic hyperplasia–a six-year experience *Eur Urol* **49**: 127.

McCullough, TC, Heldwein, FL, Soon, SJ et al. (2009) Laparoscopic versus open simple prostatectomy: an evaluation of morbidity *J Endourol* **23**: 129.

Millin T (1947) *Retropubic Urinary Surgery*. Edited by E. ES Livingstone.

Nadler RB, Blunt LW Jr, User HM et al. (2004) Preperitoneal laparoscopic simple prostatectomy *Urology* **63**: 778.

Naspro R, Suardi N, Salonia A et al. (2006) Holmium laser enucleation of the prostate versus open prostatectomy for prostates >70 g: 24-month follow-up *Eur Urol* **50**: 563.

Serretta V, Morgia G, Fondacaro L et al. (2002) Open prostatectomy for benign prostatic enlargement in southern Europe in the late 1990s: a contemporary series of 1800 interventions *Urology* **60**: 623.

Sotelo R, Clavijo R, Carmona O et al. (2008) Robotic simple prostatectomy *J Urol* **179**: 513.

Tubaro A, Carter S, Hind A et al. (2001) A prospective study of the safety and efficacy of suprapubic transvesical prostatectomy in patients with benign prostatic hyperplasia *J Urol* **166**: 172.

van Velthoven R, Peltier A, Laguna MP et al. (2004) Laparoscopic extraperitoneal adenomectomy (Millin): pilot study on feasibility *Eur Urol* **45**: 103.

Varkarakis I, Kyriakakis Z, Delis A et al. (2004) Long-term results of open transvesical prostatectomy from a contemporary series of patients *Urology* **64**: 306.

Yuh B, Laungani R, Perlmutter A et al. (2008) Robot-assisted Millin's retropubic prostatectomy: case series. *Can J Urol* **15**: 4101.

Chapter 15

Interventional treatment: transurethral resection of the prostate (TURP)

Oliver Reich and Derya Tilki

Key points

- The efficacy of conventional TURP in the improvement of subjective and objective micturitionparameters has been proven without any doubt
- While the outstanding long-term treatment efficacy of TURP is widely accepted, it was the associated morbidity of TURP which led to the development of alternative therapy modalities
- Mortalily rates with TURP are much higher in larger prostates (>60 g)
- Fewer bleeding complications and the lack of the TUR-syndrome have been repeatedly described for bipolar TURP.

15.1 Transurethral resection of the prostate (TURP)

Transurethral resection of the prostate (TURP) has been the benchmark therapy for benign prostatic hyperplasia (BPH) and for decades has been considered the reference standard of surgical treatment. This idiom in particular applies to long-term considerations, since several reports provide durable follow ups from eight to 22 years. Similar data on durability do not exist for any other instrumental BPH treatment option, including open prostatectomy (OP).

Likewise, the efficacy of TURP in improvement of subjective and objective micturition troubles, partially assessed by extensive urodynamic investigations, has been proven without any doubt (Roos et al., 1989; Zwergel et al., 1998; Madersbacher et al., 1999; Shalev et al., 1999; Wasson et al., 2000; AUA, 2003; Madersbacher et al., 2004; Varkarakis et al., 2004a; Varkarakis et al., 2004b; Madersbacher et al., 2005; Thomas et al., 2005; Berges et al., 2009).

Large-scale studies with data mostly provided by health authorities show an overall incidence of a secondary procedure associated with the initial TURP of 5.8 %, 12.3 % and 14.7 % at one, five and eight years of follow up (Roos et al., 1989; Koshiba et al., 1995; Zwergel et al., 1998; Varkarakis et al., 2004a; Madersbacher et al., 2005) These include secondary TURP, urethrotomy and bladder neck incision.

The following improvements in subjective and objective micturition parameters after 12 months have arisen from systematic meta-analyses and are described in the various guidelines:

- The International Prostate Symptom Score (IPSS) decreased by 15 to 20 (AUA, 2003; Madersbacher et al., 2004), an average reduction by 72% was calculated in an analysis of 29 randomized controlled trials (RCT) (Madersbacher et al., 1999)

- The AUA (American Urological Association) Guidelines document an average improvement in Quality of Life Score of 3.3 after 12 months (Range 0 – 6) (AUA, 2003)

- Maximum Flow rate (Qmax) improves by 10–11 ml/s within the same follow up (Roos, 1989; Shalev et al., 1999; AUA, 2003; Madersbacher et al., 2004; Varkarakis et al., 2004a; Varkarakis et al., 2004b; Madersbacher et al., 2005; Thomas et al., 2005), or relatively by 120% (Madersbacher et al., 1999). Despite its controversial significance in LUTS, a post-void residual can be reduced by 70% with TURP (Madersbacher et al., 1999).

> While the outstanding long-term treatment efficacy of TURP is widely accepted, it was the associated morbidity of TURP which led to the development of alternative therapy modalities.

A main aspect in this regard is the complication of intra- and postoperative bleeding. Perioperative transfusion rates of less than 1% have been reported in some small, single-centre series (centres of excellence). In contrast, meta-analyses have shown average perioperative transfusion rates of 8.6% for TURP (Madersbacher et al., 1999). In a large scale evaluation comprising 44 urological departments in Bavaria with data including more than 10,000 patients the transfusion rate was 2.9% (Reich et al., 2008). However, the transfusion rate and clinical relevant absorbtionsyndrom increased dramatically in prostates larger than 60 g (Reich et al., 2008).

Table 15.1 Influence of resection weight on morbidity and mortality				
Resected weight (g)	Transfusion (%)	TUR-syndrome	Revision	Mortality
< 30 g (n=5506)	2.0	1.2	5.2	0.09
30–60 g (n=3130)	3.4	1.4	6.2	0.06
> 60 g (n=561)	9.5	3.0	9.8	0.71

Alongside the perioperative bleeding, TUR syndrome, the absorption of irrigation fluid, is a seldom but potentially fatal complication of TURP. Depending on detection mode, rates vary among 0 and 7% (Roos et al., 1989; Koshiba et al., 1995; Zwergel et al., 1998; Shalev et al., 1999; Varkarakis et al., 2004a; Varkarakis et al., 2004b; Madersbacher et al., 2005; Thomas et al., 2005; Reich et al., 2008). However, a clinically relevant TUR syndrome with necessary intervention is very rare.

In addition, the AUA Guidelines (AUA, 2003)document the following relevant complications of TURP (range; 95% confidence interval):

- Post-void residual urine 5% (4–8)
- Urethral stricture/bladder neck contractures 7% (5–8)
- Cardiovascular adverse events 2% (0–6)
- Thrombembolic events 2% (0–8)
- Hematuria 6% (5–8)
- Urinary incontinence 3% (2–5)
- Urinary tract infections 6% (5–9)
- Irritative voiding symptoms 15% (9–23)
- Ejaculatory dysfunction 65% (56–72)
- Sexual dysfunction 10% (7–13).

While mortality was 2.5% 40 years ago, contemporary series show mortality rates of less than 0.10 to 0.25% (Holtgrewe et al., 1962; Horninger et al., 1996; Holman et al., 1999; Reich et al, 2008). However, mortality rates with TURP are much higher in prostates larger than 60 g compared to prostates smaller than 60 g (Table 15.1) (Reich et al., 2008).

The described relevant spectrum of complications of TURP and emerging competing minimally invasive laser procedures have led to different modifications and innovations in transurethral high-frequency surgery. These consist of advancements in high-frequency generators such as the so-called "coagulant intermittent cutting" (CIC), which led to a reduction of rates of transfusion and TUR syndrome. Similar modulations of the high frequency generators such as dry-cut resection are already in clinical use (Alschibaja et al., 2005).

On the other hand, modulations of the electrode are critical innovations. However, these cause changes in the high-frequency current. Because these techniques (*bipolar resection* in isotonic irrigation fluid with bipolar resection device, *plasma vaporization* of the prostate) differ significantly from conventional TURP, these are discussed in separate chapters.

15.1.1 Transurethral incision of the prostate (TUIP)

Transurethral Incision of the prostate (TUIP) can be recommended for young, sexually active men with a prostate volume of less than 30 ml (Berges et al., 2009). Several randomized trials have reported a comparable efficacy of TUIP in comparison to TURP for this patient population (Madersbacher et al., 1999). In a meta-analysis of six randomized clinical trials comparing TUIP with TURP with a follow up of more than six months, Madersbacher et al. conclude that efficacy of TUIP in that subgroup is comparable or slightly inferior to TURP (Madersbacher et al., 1999).

Nonetheless, re-intervention rates were clearly favourable for TURP compared to TUIP (2.6 % vs. 15.9 %). Concerning morbidity however, TUIP provided superior results in terms of blood transfusions (TUIP: 0.4 % vs. TURP: 8.6 %) and retrograde ejaculation (TUIP: 18.2 % vs. TURP: 65.4 %).

For the appropriate patient TUIP is recommended in the EAU and AUA guidelines on BPH (AUA, 2003; Madersbacher et al., 2004; Berges et al., 2009). Given the portion of 84.8% for TURP and 2.4% for TUIP of instrumental BPS therapy in Germany 2004 (Yang et al., 2001; Alschibaja et al., 2005), some urologists believe that TUIP is an underutilized technique. However, candidates for TUIP form a selected patient group (Yang et al. 2001).

15.2 Transurethral bipolar resection of the prostate

Bleeding complications and TUR syndrome of conventional monopolarTURP have been the main reasons for the advancement of the gold standard TURP. Changes of the electrodes and the high-frequency generators have contributed significantly to improved hemostasis of modern TURP.

In contrast to monopolar systems, bipolar TURP uses high-frequency electric current flowing between two electrodes within the surgical instrument. The major advantage of bipolar resection over the conventional monopolar technique, in which the current flows through the tissue, is the use of isotonic irrigation fluid eliminating the possibility of TUR syndrome (hypotonic hyperhydration with hyponatremia).

Different contradictory data regarding comparisons of monopolar and bipolar TURP exist. In a recent systematic meta-analysis of 16 randomized controlled trials (RCTs) no clinically relevant differences in short-term efficacy (after 12 months) have been found between monopolar and bipolar TURP (Mamoulakis et al., 2009).

Furthermore, no differences were evident regarding operation time and rates of adverse events such as transfusions, retention after catheter removal, or urethral complications. However, bipolar TURP was found to be preferable due to a more favourable safety profile (lower TUR syndrome and clot retention rates) and shorter irrigation and catheterization duration. The authors conclude that well-designed multicentric/international RCTs with long-term follow-up and cost analysis are still needed.

Less bleeding complications and improved hemostasis have been repeatedly described for bipolar TURP in literature (Dunsmuir et al., 2003; Starkman et al., 2005; Tefekli et al., 2005; de Autorino et al., 2006). However, these observations are not supported by objective criteria such as postoperative change in hb-level and transfusion rates (Fung et al., 2005; de Autorino et al., 2006; Reich et al., 2008). Nevertheless, other criteria such as irrigation volume and mean catherization time seem to support the use of bipolar TURP (Mamoulakis et al., 2009). Data from international RCTs with long-term follow-up (>12 mo) remain to be awaited.

15.3 Bipolar plasma vaporization of the prostate

Bipolar plasma vaporization technique was introduced in 2008 (Reich et al., 2009). This method was developed in an attempt to combine the benefits of vaporization techniques (good hemostasis, low morbidity, low learning curve because of easy handling) and bipolar resection. It derives from plasmakinetic bipolar resection of the prostate and utilizes well-known electrical principles.

The instrument consists of a bipolar mushroom-like electrode (Reich et al., 2009). Plasma vaporization of the prostate is performed under direct visualization using the electrode in a near-contact technique (hoovering technique).

Monopolar electrovaporization of the prostate, which was performed using a rollerball electrode, has been abandoned due to the disproportionate extent of coagulation (up to 10 mm) in the tissue treated, leading to mostly irritative side-effects and stress incontinence.

The coagulation extent is much lower in bipolar plasma vaporization and the initial results are promising (Reich et al., 2009). Because of the wide availability of bipolar high-frequency generators and a comparable low learning curve, this technique has found broad clinical use. Longer follow-up is to be awaited before definite conclusions can be drawn.

References

Alschibaja M, May F, Treiber U et al. (2005) Transurethral resection for benign prostatic hyperplasia. current developments *Urologe A* **44**: 499.

AUA guideline on management of benign prostatic hyperplasia (2003) Chapter 1: Diagnosis and treatment recommendations *J Urol* **170**: 530.

Berges R, Dreikorn K, Hofner K et al. (2009) [Diagnostic and differential diagnosis of benign prostate syndrome (BPS): Guidelines of the German Urologists] *Urologe A*.

de Autorino R, Quarto G et al. Gyrus bipolar versus standard monopolar transurethral resection of the prostate: a randomized prospective trial *Urology* **67**: 69.

Dunsmuir WD, McFarlane JP, Tan A et al. (2003) Gyrus bipolar electrovaporization vs transurethral resection of the prostate: a randomized prospective single-blind trial with 1 y follow-up *Prostate Cancer Prostatic Dis* **6**: 182.

Fung BT, Li SK, Yu CF et al. (2005) Prospective randomized controlled trial comparing plasmakinetic vaporesection and conventional transurethral resection of the prostate *Asian J Surg* **28**: 24.

Holman CD, Wisniewski ZS, Semmens JB et al. (1999) Mortality and prostate cancer risk in 19,598 men after surgery for benign prostatic hyperplasia *BJU Int* **84**: 37.

Holtgrewe HL, Valk WL (1962) Factors influencing the mortality and morbidity of transurethral prostatectomy: a study of 2,015 cases *J Urol* **87**: 450.

Horninger W, Unterlechner H, Strasser H et al. (1996) Transurethral prostatectomy: mortality and morbidity. *Prostate* **28**: 195.

Koshiba K, Egawa S, Ohori M et al. Does transurethral resection of the prostate pose a risk to life? 22-year outcome *J Urol* **153**: 1506.

Madersbacher S, Alivizatos G, Nordling, J et al. (2004) EAU 2004 guidelines on assessment, therapy and follow-up of men with lower urinary tract symptoms suggestive of benign prostatic obstruction (BPH guidelines) *Eur Urol* **46**: 547.

Madersbacher S, Lackner J, Brossner C et al. (2005) Reoperation, myocardial infarction and mortality after transurethral and open prostatectomy: a nation-wide, long-term analysis of 23,123 cases *Eur Urol* **47**: 499.

Madersbacher S, Marberger M (1999) Is transurethral resection of the prostate still justified? *BJU Int* **83**: 227.

Reich O, Gratzke C, Bachmann A et al. (2008) Morbidity, mortality and early outcome of transurethral resection of the prostate: a prospective multicenter evaluation of 10,654 patients *J Urol* **180**: 246.

Reich O, Schenker B, Gratzke C et al. (2009) Plasma vaporisation of the prostate: initial clinical results *Eur Urol*.

Mamoulakis C, Ubbink DT, de la Rosette JJ. (2009) Bipolar versus monopolar transurethral resection of the prostate: a systematic review and meta-analysis of randomized controlled trials *Eur Urol*.

Roos NP, Wennberg JE, Malenka DJ et al. (1989) Mortality and reoperation after open and transurethral resection of the prostate for benign prostatic hyperplasia *N Engl J Med* **320**: 1120.

Shalev M, Richter S, Kessler O et al. (1999) Long-term incidence of acute myocardial infarction after open and transurethral resection of the prostate for benign prostatic hyperplasia *J Urol* **161**: 491.

Starkman JS, Santucci RA (2005) Comparison of bipolar transurethral resection of the prostate with standard transurethral prostatectomy: shorter stay, earlier catheter removal and fewer complications *BJU Int* **95**: 69.

Tefekli A, Muslumanoglu AY, Baykal M et al. (2005) A hybrid technique using bipolar energy in transurethral prostate surgery: a prospective, randomized comparison *J Urol* **174**: 1339.

Thomas AW, Cannon A, Bartlett E et al. (2005) The natural history of lower urinary tract dysfunction in men: minimum 10-year urodynamic followup of transurethral resection of prostate for bladder outlet obstruction *J Urol* **174**: 1887.

Varkarakis I, Kyriakakis Z, Delis A et al. (2004a) Long-term results of open transvesical prostatectomy from a contemporary series of patients *Urology*, **64**: 306.

Varkarakis J, Bartsch G, Horninger W (2004b) Long-term morbidity and mortality of transurethral prostatectomy: a 10-year follow-up *Prostate* **58**: 248.

Wasson JH, Bubolz TA, Lu-Yao GL et al. (2000) Transurethral resection of the prostate among medicare beneficiaries: 1984 to 1997. For the Patient Outcomes Research Team for Prostatic Diseases *J Urol* **164**: 1212.

Yang Q, Peters TJ, Donovan JL et al. (2001) Transurethral incision compared with transurethral resection of the prostate for bladder outlet obstruction: a systematic review and meta-analysis of randomized controlled trials *J Urol* **165**: 1526.

Zwergel U, Wullich B, Lindenmeir U et al. (1998) Long-term results following transurethral resection of the prostate *Eur Urol* **33**: 476.

Chapter 16

Interventional treatment: Prostate laser

Thomas Hermanns and Tullio Sulser

> **Key points**
>
> - Lasers for BPH treatment attracted the attention of urologists due to excellent tissue ablative and haemostatic properties
> - Several lasers with different properties and application devices have been developed
> - Laser procedures are the most extensively investigated minimal invasive BPH treatments
> - Lasers with pure coagulative properties caused considerable postoperative dysuria and prolonged urinary retention and are no longer in use
> - Haemostatic properties allow for treatment of patients under full anticoagulation or dual platelet aggregation inhibition.

16.1 History of prostate laser surgery

The introduction of transurethral electroresection of the prostate (TURP) for the treatment of benign prostatic hyperplasia (BPH) in the mid 20th century represented a major advance over open surgical prostatic enucleation. The endoscopic technique soon became the new gold standard for prostatic deobstruction.

However, a significant morbidity of TURP (i.e. bleeding with clot retention or transfusion and TUR-syndrome) and the wish to perform an effective office procedure mainly prompted the development of less invasive alternative procedures.

In the past 25 years, several new technologies (i.e. stents, dilatation balloons, lasers, focused ultrasound, microwave, and radiofrequency devices) have been experimentally and clinically evaluated.

Of these technologies, the laser procedures were and still are the most extensively investigated.

Coagulation of superficial tumours of the urinary bladder and the outer genitalia were the earliest successfully performed urologic laser procedures. The first laser application to the prostate was reported in 1979 by Böwering et al. who performed laser-coagulation of the prostatic cavity after TURP in patients with prostate cancer.

In 1985, Shanberg et al. investigated laser prostatomy in small prostates, a technique that never became widely accepted. Major progression in pure laser therapy of BPH was made at the beginning of the 1990s. Not only different lasers with their specific wavelengths and tissue penetration properties but also different applications with special laser fibres and various power settings for different methods of ablation (coagulation, incision, vaporization, resection, and enucleation) were evaluated.

16.2 Neodymium: Yttrium-Aluminium-Garnet (Nd:YAG) lasers

Low-powered (40 W) Nd:YAG laser coagulation was the first laser procedure used for prostatic de-obstruction. In the late 1990s higher power settings were also used in order to vaporize the obstructive tissue. In the early years several ablative techniques were developed.

> The good tissue penetratin properties of the low powered laser resulted in deep coagulation necrosis of the adenoma which subsequently sloughed off and passed through the urethra over the following weeks.

The first experimental report of a transurethral ultrasound-guided laser prostatectomy (TULIP) appeared in 1991, and soon clinical experience was reported by different groups. The TULIP probe contained a 90° laser port to emit the laser beam, an ultrasound transducer to control the procedure and a laser-transparent balloon to fix the device in the prostatic urethra. Following several reports of substantial improvements in subjective and objective outcome, TULIP was soon abandoned. The difficult performance of the procedure, the need for prolonged postoperative catheterization and persisting irritative voiding symptoms were the main reasons for its failure.

Visually assisted laser prostatectomy (VLAP) with a user-friendly non-contact side-firing fibre markedly raised the popularity of BPH laser treatment. Costello et al. were among the first who reported VLAP in 1992. Although VLAP resulted in considerable improvements in symptoms and was associated with low morbidity, prolonged dysuria and catheter depending urinary retention were often bothersome for the patients. An associated high re-operation rate up to 15% within the first three years and poor functional long-term results caused that VLAP has been abandoned.

To overcome the problem of prolonged catheterization Nd:YAG contact laser ablation of the prostate (CLAP) with special sapphire-tipped fibres converting laser energy into heat was developed. Very high temperatures at the tip of the fibre which was placed in direct contact to the surface resulted in tissue vaporization with immediate debulking. Hence, urinary retention and perturbing dysuria were rarer.

However, slow and tedious tissue ablation limited this procedure to only small sized prostates. CLAP did not establish itself as a viable alternative procedure due to the lack of substantial improvements of the system and high re-operation rates up to 43% after five years.

Interstitial laser coagulation (ILC) which was first reported by Muschter in 1995 was another technique mainly developed to overcome postoperative problems known from early Nd:YAG laser applications. Special laser fibres were placed into the obstructing adenoma. Application of laser energy for several minutes resulted in tissue coagulation along the distal millimeters of the fibre. Sparing of the urethral mucosa reduced prolonged tissue sloughing with irritative voiding symptoms. However, re-catheterization, moderate functional results and high re-treatment rates up to 40% within three years were the reasons why ILC failed as alternative procedure.

16.3 **Diode lasers**

The first experience with the diode laser occurred in the late 1990s with the indigo-diode laser system which was used for ILC. The technique did not gain wide acceptance due to comparable results and drawbacks known from Nd:YAG ILC. More recently, diode laser vaporization systems with high power settings up to 200 W have been experimentally and clinically evaluated. The main advantages of this laser system are the low costs of the laser and a high power output caused by more efficient diode laser light beam amplification (so-called pumping) compared to lasers using Arc lamp pumping.

16.4 **Prostate lasers in 2011**

The drawbacks of Nd:YAG laser treatment led to the development of novel laser systems with different properties. Once it was realized that immediate tissue ablation is important, other wavelengths were evaluated for prostate surgery.

Vaporization or resection of the prostate using the high power Holmium:YAG laser (HoLRP) was very time consuming and showed only moderate success. The well evaluated Holmium laser enucleation (HoLEP) technique, however, has been shown to be equivalent or even superior to TURP in terms of functional outcome and overall complication rate. A considerable learning curve and the need for tedious tissue morcelation after enucleation are the main reasons why a widespread use of HoLEP failed to appear.

The Thulium:YAG laser is another newer-generation laser which can be used for either vaporesection or enucleation of the prostate. Long-term results, which are still lacking, are expected to be equivalent to those following HoLEP.

Halving the wavelength of the Nd:YAG laser from 1064 nm to 532 nm by interposition of potassium-titanyl-phosphate (KTP) or lithium triborat (LBO) crystals, not only results in the emission of green laser light but also in completely different laser tissue interaction including improved vaporization and reduced coagulation of the prostatic tissue.

The KTP-Greenlight laser vaporization was introduced in 1998 by Malek et al. To increase the efficacy of the procedure, elevation of the power output from initially 30 W to 120 W and modifications of the laser beam by replacing the KTP crystal by a LBO crystal have been performed over the last decade. The well evaluated Greenlight laser procedure has to be considered as reference standard for laser vaporization of the prostate. Furthermore, the technique is particularly suitable for patients under antiplatelet or anticoagulation therapy due to excellent haemostatic properties.

In 2011, only Ho:YAG and 532nm-Greenlight laser prostatectomy have shown evidence of safety and effectiveness. Especially for Ho:LEP, available long-term data provide an equivalent, or even superior outcome compared to TURP as well as high-level evidence of durability.

Many of the early laser systems did not challenge the status quo for a long time and were abandoned mainly due to prolonged postoperative dysuria, the need for post-operative catheterization and high re-operation rates. However, the step-by-step understanding of laser tissue interactions and their specific drawbacks led to modifications which substantially improved BPH laser treatments over the years. Only if a laser system can provide easy handling, improved safety, adequate costs, and efficiency comparable to TURP, will it supersede TURP as the so-called golden standard in BPH surgery.

References

Böwering R, Hofstetter A, Keiditsch E, Frank F (1979) Irradiation of prostatic carcinoma by neodymium-YAG-laser. In: Optics and photonics applied to medicine *SPIE Proc* **211**: 16–20.

Costello AJ, Bowsher WG, Bolton DM, Braslis KG, Burt J (1992) Laser ablation of the prostate in patients with benign prostatic hypertrophy. *Br J Urol.* **69**(6): 603–8.

Dixon CM (1995) Lasers for the treatment of benign prostatic hyperplasia *Urol Clin North Am* **22**(2): 413–22.

Kabalin JN (1995) Laser coagulation prostatectomy: evolution of clinical practice and treatment parameters *J Endourol.* **9**(2): 93–9.

Malek RS, Barrett DM, Kuntzman RS (1998) High-power potassium-titanyl-phosphate (KTP/532) laser vaporization prostatectomy: 24 hours later *Urology* **51**(2): 254–6.

Muschter R, Zellner M, Hessel S, Hofstetter A (1995) Interstitial laser-induced coagulation of the prostate for therapy of benign hyperplasia *Urologe A* **34**(2): 90–7.

Naspro R, Salonia A, Colombo R, Cestari A, Guazzoni G, Rigatti P, Montorsi F (2005) Update of the minimally invasive therapies for benign prostatic hyperplasia *Curr Opin Urol* **15**(1): 49–53.

Roth RA, Aretz HT (1991) Transurethral ultrasound-guided laser-induced prostatectomy (TULIP procedure): a canine prostate feasibility study *J Urol.* **146**(4): 1128–35.

Shanberg AM, Tansey LA, and Baghdassarian R (1985) The use of the neodymium YAG laser in prostatotomy *J Urol* **133**: 196A.

te Slaa E, de la Rosette JJ (1996) Lasers in the treatment of benign prostatic obstruction: past, present, and future *Eur Urol.* **30**(1): 1–10.

Chapter 17

Interventional treatment: Greenlight laser

Malte Riethen and Alexander Bachmann

> **Key points**
>
> - Greenlight laser vaporization is characterized by TUR-like technique and a short learning curve
> - The physical properties of the 532 nm based laser result in a virtually bloodless and safe procedure
> - Surgery can also be performed by experienced surgeons safe and effective in patients with platelet inhibition therapy or oral anticoagulation
> - Length of catheterization and hospitalization are shorter than with TURP
> - Short- and intermediate term results are comparable to TURP.

17.1 Background

In the early 1990s visual laser ablation of the prostate with the 1064 nm Neodymium:Yttrium-Aluminium-Garnet (Nd:YAG) laser was introduced. The laser had a very low absorption coefficient in most tissues so that is penetrates tissue deeply between 4 and 18 mm. The energy density in the tissue was low, which resulted in a deep coagulative necrosis of the tissue. Although VLAP significantly reduced the need for blood transfusions, improvement of symptoms and voiding parameters was inferior to TURP and the rate of reoperations was considerably higher. Thus, VLAP has largely been abandoned.

By passing the Nd:YAG-produced beam through a KTP (Greenlight PV) or LBO (Greenligth HPS) crystal, a green visible light beam of

532 nm, which has a completely different laser beam, tissue interaction is generated. The first laser models used a 60 W generator, which showed only a slow ablation of the tissue. By increasing the power of the laser to 80 W and later to 120 W efficient ablation could be achieved. In 2010 the 180 Watts powered Xcellerated Performers System (XPS) including a new Fiber technique was launched. However, data not available in 2010.

17.2 **The physical properties of the Greenlight laser**

Laser light comprises a single wavelength of collimated light, which is emitted by a laser source. When this light passes though the tissue energy is converted to heat.

Since the densitiy of energy delivered to the tissue is low, heating remains below the boiling temperature, causing coagulation, but not vaporization. In contrast, the 532 nm based KTP or LBO-laser energy is strongly absorbed by haemoglobin and penetrates tissue only to a depth of 3 mm.

The limited depth of penetration leads to a high power density inside superficial tissue layers causing a rapid vaporization of the tissue, giving the technique its name, photoselective vaporization of the prostate (PVP). Only a limited quantity of energy penetrates deeper, so that a 2 mm rim of coagulated tissue remains in the underlying tissue. The physical properties of the 80 W and 120 W laser have been studied extensively in experimental settings demonstrating more efficient vaporisation at higher power levels and a thin coagulation zone.

17.3 **Operative technique**

The operative technique of PVP consists of various steps:
- After introduction of the cystoscope, which has a separation for the laser fibre and the irrigation solution, a cystoscopy is performed to visualize the ureteral orifices
- The procedure is started at the bladder neck or the median lobe under vision in a free beam fibre-sweeping technique. The recommended distance to the surface is about 0.5 mm, providing an optimal energy delivery to the tissue and a maximum vaporization effect, demonstrated by a visible bubble formation

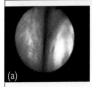
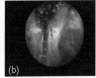
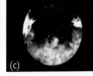

(a) (b) (c)

From: Bachmann et al. (2005) Photoselective vaporization (PVP) versus transurethral
resection of the prostate (TURP): a prospective bi-centre study of perioperative morbidity
and early functional outcome *Eur Urology* **48**,: 965–972 © Elsevier.

- The vaporization is continued from the neck of the bladder to
the apex of the prostate; therefore the fibre is slowly rotated
between the thumb and the index finger and moved anterior
and posterior
- Afterwards, the lateral lobes, the apex and the bladder neck
are vaporized. If bleeding occurs, coagulation can be induced
by moving the fibre 3 to 4 mm from the tissue. Coagulation for
haemostasis should be conducted at low power
- At the end of the procedure, a real prostatic cavity should be
visible (Figure 17.1)
- Disadvantages of GreenLight: Energy limitation of fibre to
275 kJ in GreenLight PV and GreenLight HPS. With introducing
"MoJo" (more Joule), energy application is possible up to
400 kJ per fibre.

Recently, in 2010 the new XPS-Generation of GreenLight laser
(AMS™) was introduced in order to overcome the disadvantage
of insufficient tissue removal in larger prostates providing higher
output up to 180 W, a larger vaporization area and a so called
non-degradable laser fibre (MoXy), including a contact-stop
modus which will preserve the tip of the fiber from destruction
because of reflection. Clinical data are awaited.

17.4 Clinical outcomes of photoselective vaporization of the prostate

One of the major advantages of PVP is the relatively short learning
curve and the low rate of intra- and perioperative complications.
Several studies have proven the high intraoperative safety of PVP

alone or in comparison to TURP or OP and in subgroups of patients with large prostates, on anticoagulation or in retention:

- In an analysis of 500 patients undergoing 80 W KTP PVP intra-operative bleeding was reported in 3.6%, capsule perforation in 0.2% and conversion to TURP due to bleeding, prostate size or fibre defect in 5.2% of the patients. No TUR-syndrome was observed and no blood transfusions were necessary

The high intraoperative safety could be confirmed for the 120 W LBO-laser:

- The analysis of intraoperative complication of patients on anticoagulation, on retention or with prostates larger than 80 to 100 ml showed no significant difference to the average population of patients

The randomized study comparing 80-W PVP with OP for prostates greater than 80 ml could confirm the safety of the method:

- Significantly higher rate of perioperative blood transfusions in the OP group
- No difference in the incidence of postoperative complications
- In comparison to TURP, the rate of blood transfusions, the length of catheterization and the duration of hospital stay are significantly lower.

Postoperative bladder storage symptoms and urge incontinence are usually self-limiting within the first three months after surgery and can effectively be treated with anti-inflammatory drugs, antibiotic therapy or anti-muscarinic drugs. The rate is usually higher than after standard TURP, patients with history of chronic prostatitis tend to suffer from postoperative storage symptoms more frequently.

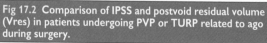

Fig 17.2 Comparison of IPSS and postvoid residual volume (Vres) in patients undergoing PVP or TURP related to ago during surgery.

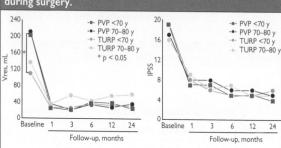

From: Ruszat et al. (2008) Comparison of potassium-titanyl-phosphate laser vaporization of the prostate and transurethral resection of the prostate: update of a prospective non-randomized two-centre study *BJU Intl* **102**: 1432–9 © John Wiley & Sons 2008.

A limitation in the evaluation of the longevity of PVP is the current lack of long-term data from randomized trials. The longest follow-up with the highest number of patients was reported by Hai:

• Of 246 patients available for analysis at 5-year follow-up after PVP, 19 had to be retreated with PVP due to recurrent adenoma and three underwent incision of the bladder neck resulting in an overall retreatment rate of 8.9%

• Symptom score, quality of life, peak flow rate, postvoid residue volume and PSA showed a significant improvement as compared to the preoperative level.

These data are comparable with results from other centres analyzing 500 patients:

• Voiding symptoms and micturition parameters showed a significant improvement.

• Anticoagulation and urinary retention at the time of surgery have no significant influence on the rate of long-term complications and clinical outcome.

Results from a randomized trial comparing PVP and TURP shows no significant difference in terms of obstruction relief, whereas a randomized trial in larger prostates (>70 ml) found better functional results at six-months control in the TURP arm. Comparing OP to 80-W PVP, no difference was found regarding late morbidity, however longer follow-up needs to be awaited taking an observation period of only 18 months into account. The impact of PVP on male sexual function has been studied rarely. Existing evidence suggests a general improvement of erectile dysfunction related to lower urinary tract symptoms.

In summary PVP offers a safe and effective treatment alternative to TURP in patients with symptomatic prostate enlargement and should especially taken into consideration in patients with high risk of bleeding.

Table 17.1 Comparison of TURP and PVP		
	TURP	**PVP**
Short learning curve	yes	yes
Surgery in patients with ongoing anticoagulation	no	yes
Surgery in larger prostates (>80 to 100 ml)	no	yes
Tissue for histopathologic evaluation	yes	no
Risk of TUR-Syndrome	yes	no
Long-term results	yes	no

References

Choi B, Tabatabaei S, Bachmann A, Collins E, de la Rosette J, Gomez Sancha F, Muir G, Reich O, Woo H (2008) GreenLight HPS 120-W laser for benign prostatic hyperplasia: comparative complications and technical recommendations *Eur Urol Suppl* **7**(4): 384–92.

Hai, M. (2009) Photoselective vaporization of prostate: five-year outcomes of entire clinic patient population *Urology* **73**(4): 807–10.

Horasanli K, Silay MS, Altay B, Tanriverdi O, Sarica K, Miroglu C. (2008) Photoselective potassium titanyl phosphate (KTP) laser vaporization versus transurethral resection of the prostate for prostates larger than 70 mL: a short-term prospective randomized trial *Urology* **71**(2): 247–51.

Naspro R, Bachmann A, Gilling P, Kuntz R, Madersbacher S, Montorsi F, Reich O, Stief C, Vavassori I (2009) A review of the recent evidence (2006–2008) for 532-nm photoselective laser vaporisation and Holmium laser enucleation of the prostate *Eur Urol* **55**: 1345–57.

De la Rosette J, Collins E, Bachmann A, Choi B, Muir G, Reich O, Gomez Sancha F, Tabatabaei S, Woo H (2008) Historical aspects of laser therapy for benign prostatic hyperplasia *Eur Urol Suppl* **7**(4): 363–9.

Ruszat R, Seitz M, Wyler SF, Abe C, Rieken M, Reich O, Gasser TC, Bachmann A. (2008) GreenLight laser vaporization of the prostate: single-center experience and long-term results after 500 procedures *Eur Urol* **54**(4): 893–901.

Woo H, Reich O, Bachmann A, Choi B, Collins E, de la Rosette J, Gomez Sancha F, Muir G, Tabatabaei S (2008) Outcome of the GreenLight HPS 120-W laser therapy in specific patient populations: those in retention, on anticoagulants, and with large prostates (≥ 80 ml) *Eur Urol Suppl* **7**(4): 378–83.

Chapter 18

Interventional treatment: Holmium laser

Liam C. Wilson and Peter J. Gilling

Key points

- The Holmium laser has excellent haemostatic and incisional properties
- Patients having Holmium laser enucleation of the Prostate have:
  - Reduced perioperative morbidity, catheter time and hospital stay when compared to TURP or open prostatectomy
  - Equivalent subjective and objective outcomes when compared to TURP or open prostatectomy
  - Wide applicability—no limit to the size of the prostate that can be treated.

Transurethral Resection of the Prostate (TURP) has long been the operation of choice for the surgical treatment of men with benign prostatic hyperplasia (BPH). However, alternative, minimally invasive treatments have been sought which attempt to reduce perioperative morbidity when compared to TURP, while having at least an equivalent clinical effect. Holmium laser enucleation of the prostate (HoLEP) remains the only alternative treatment that removes more prostatic tissue than TURP, while having less perioperative morbidity and equivalent or better outcomes than TURP.

18.1 Holmium laser

The key properties of the Holmium laser that make it such a successful instrument for prostatic surgery are:

- The wavelength (2140nm) creates an energy density high enough to create precise cutting and incision, while the dissipating heat and coagulating small and medium sized vessels

- The pulsed nature of this laser aids in its ability to safely dissect in the surgical planes of the prostate
- Normal Saline is used as the operative irrigant, avoiding the risk of the Transurethral (TUR) Syndrome which can occur with TURP
- The enucleated tissue has to be removed by transurethral resection of morcellation.

18.2 Holmium Laser Enucleation of Prostate (HoLEP)

The surgical indications for HoLEP are identical to those for TURP. In addition, HoLEP can be safely performed on anticoagulated patients, which is not possible with TURP.

The procedure itself involves the retrograde enucleation of the three lobes of the prostate. The laser is introduced via a laser resectoscope, and is sheathed inside a 6F ureteric catheter. The anatomical landmarks are the veru montanum, the prostatic capsule and the bladder neck. Two bladder neck incisions are made at 5 and 7 o'clock, from the bladder neck to the veru, to define the median lobe. A single incision is often employed if the median lobe is small. The lobe is then dissected off the capsule, working proximally, where it is released at the level of the bladder neck. The pane of dissection is easily identified as the prostatic capsule has transverse running fibres. The lateral lobes are similarly enucleated, using the previously made bladder neck incisions, and an incision made superiorly at the 12 o'clock position.

Haemostasis is achieved by "defocusing" the laser, which occurs by bringing the laser fibre away from contact with the tissue which coagulates rather than vaporises tissue. Once enucleation has been completed, the resectoscope is replaced with a long nephroscope(through a common sheath), which allows the soft tissue morcellator to be introduced into the bladder. The morcelator uses reciprocating blades to reduce the prostatic lobes into small fragments which are then removed by high power suction. This is performed with the bladder distended, and good visibility is essential.

Unlike TURP, which has significant risks of TUR Syndrome if the procedure is prolonged (>60 minutes), there is no such restriction for HoLEP, and therefore any size of prostate can be treated. The largest prostate treated in our institution is 1100g. The properties of the laser mean that 95% of patients do not require continuous bladder irrigation after TURP, and usually a 20F 2 way indwelling catheter (IDC) is placed. 90% of men are discharged within 24 hours of surgery.

18.3 **HoLEP Vs TURP**

HoLEP, unlike many alternative treatments for BPH, is a well studied treatment, and well designed randomised controlled trials comparing HoLEP to TURP have showed that those patients having HoLEP have:

- Reduced catheter time
- Reduced perioperative complications
- Reduced hospital stay
- Equivalent outcomes regarding symptomatic improvement (IPSS scores) and urinary flow rates (Qmax) and superior urodynamic findings.

Unlike TURP, (where blood transfusion rates are as high as 5%), transfusions are rare after HoLEP. There were no transfusions in the HoLEP group of the three randomized trials. In our unit, the transfusion rate is approximately 1 in 3,000 cases. The need for postoperative reintervention for recurrent BPH is 1% at 6 years. Bladder mucosal injury caused by the morcellator is a complication unique to HoLEP/morcellation, but in the vast majority of cases is minor and does not affect the post-operative course.

While HoLEP is often slower than TURP in treating small-moderate sized glands, significantly more prostate tissue is removed with HoLEP and therefore the efficiency of the operation is equivalent to TURP.

> As prostate volume increases, HoLEP becomes significantly more efficient than TURP, and in very large glands, HoLEP needs to be compared with open prostatectomy.

Several studies have shown that the reduction in PSA after treatment correlates well with the amount of adenoma resected. This is important indirect evidence to consider when comparing established techniques such as TURP and HoLEP with non-ablative techniques such as the Diode or Nd:YAG lasers, where no tissue is removed. After HoLEP, PSA commonly drops by 81–86%, or by 90%. In contrast, PSA levels after ablative techniques will only reduce by 30–40%.

Delayed morbidity for HoLEP is low and not significantly different from TURP morbidity. A pooled analysis of over 1,800 patients demonstrated that incontinence occurred in 1.1% of patients, urethral stricture in 1.9% of patients and bladder neck contracture in 1.5%.

With respect to sexual function, there is no difference in outcome between TURP and HoLEP. Due to the fact that the bladder neck is incised, both TURP and HoLEP commonly cause retrograde ejaculation, but erectile dysfunction is rare.

Comparative and long-term results after HoLEP available with level 1a evidence.

While the favourable perioperative outcomes for HoLEP made it a popular surgical treatment for BPH initially, its popularity may be cemented by its durability. Prostatic regrowth occurs after any surgical technique, but the fact that whole lobes of the prostate are removed at HoLEP means that this risk is minimized.

Conversely, the technique at highest risk of prostatic regrowth causing recurrence of symptoms is ablation. Again, the durability of HoLEP has been well studied (unlike many other minimally invasive techniques) and studies 2-7 years post-operatively have confirmed a sustained clinical benefit, as well as a very low re-operation rate.

18.4 **HoLEP vs open prostatectomy**

As there is no size limit to the prostate that can be treated by HoLEP, the comparison for larger prostates is between HoLEP and open prostatectomy (OP). Blood loss, blood transfusion rates and hospital stay are significantly lower for HoLEP. There is no difference in the amount of prostatic tissue removed between the two techniques, or in the patient's symptomatic outcomes between the two techniques, and the durability of clinical effect has been confirmed.

As prostate volume increases, HoLEP becomes significantly more efficient than TURP, and in very large glands, HoLEP needs to be compared with open prostatectomy.

18.5 **HoLEP and the learning curve**

One of the commonly described reasons that HoLEP has not become more popular is the "learning curve". There is no doubt that some training and mentoring is required, but there are some advantages to learning HoLEP over TURP. As there is no risk of TUR syndrome and haemostasis is easier to achieve, there is less restriction of vision and no operative time constraints as there is for TURP.

Dissection in the surgical plane between adenoma and capsule is also conceptually easier for novices. Studies have shown that approximately 20 cases are required to achieve competence. Although good outcomes are achieved early in the operative series, enucleation efficiency improves with time. Other studies demonstrate that results equivalent to published experts can be achieved after 50 cases. When learning HoLEP, a short intense period of instruction and mentoring is helpful, as well as careful case selection of prostates less than 60cc.

18.6 **Holmium Laser Ablation of the Prostate (HoLAP)**

Early in the evolution of Holmium prostate surgery, ablation was the only technique available, but was associated with significant post-operative irritative symptoms and lack of a durable effect. The technique was superceded by the resection (HoLRP) and then enucleation (HoLEP) procedures. However, ablative techniques have become more visible on the back of aggressive marketing campaigns. While no tissue is removed, and surgical time is prolonged, HoLAP remains an option in men with small volume prostate glands.

In several well designed randomised clinical trials, HoLEP has reduced perioperative morbidity, catheter time, and hospital stay when compared to TURP and open prostatectomy. Symptomatic improvement is at least equivalent when comparing HoLEP and TURP/open prostatectomy. HoLEP removes more prostatic tissue than TURP, and this is the reason the clinical improvement is preserved and the reoperation rate is low in the long term.

References

Aho T, Gilling P, Kennett K, Westenburg AM, Fraundorfer MR, Frampton CM (2005) Holmium laser bladder neck incision versus Holmium laser enucleation of the prostateas outpatient procedures for prostates less than 40 grams: a randomized trial *J Urol* **174**: 210–14.

Ahyai S, Kuntz R, Lehrich K (2007) Holmium laser enucleation versus transurethral resection of the prostate: 3-year follow-up results of a randomized clinical trial *Eur Urol* **52**(5): 1456–63.

El-Hakim A, Elhilali MM (2002) Holmium laser enucleation of the prostate can be taught: the first learning experience *BJU Int* **90**(9): 863–9.

Elzayat EA, Elhilali MM (2007) Holmium laser enucleation of the prostate (HoLEP): long-term results, reoperation rate, and possible impact of the learning curve *Eur Urol* **52**(5): 1465–71.

Gilling PJ (2008) Holmium laser Enucleation of the Prostate (HoLEP). Surgery Illustrated *BJUI Int.* **101**(1): 131–42.

Kuntz R, Ahyai S, Lehrich K, Fayad A (2004) Transurethral holmium laser enucleation of the prostate versus transurethral electrocautery resection of the prostate: a randomized prospective trial in 200 patients *J Urol* **172**(3): 1012–6.

Kuntz R, Ahyai S, Lehrich K (2004) Transurethral holmium laser enucleation of the prostate compared with transvesical open prostatectomy: 18-month follow-up of a randomized trial *J Endourol* **18**(2): 189–91.

Kuntz R, Lehrich K, Ahyai S (2008) Holmium laser enucleation of the prostate versus open prostatectomy for prostates greater than 100 grams: 5-year follow-up results of a randomised clinical trial *Eur Urol* **53**(1): 160–6.

Montorsi F, Naspro R, Salonia A, et al. (2008) Holmium laser enucleation versus transurethral resection of the prostate: results from a 2-center prospective randomized trial in patients with obstructive benign prostatic hyperplasia *J Urol* **179**(5): S87–90.

Tan AHH, Gilling PJ, Kennett KM, et al. (2003) Randomized trial comparing Holmium laser enucleation of prostate with transurethral resection of prostate for treatment of bladder outlet obstruction secondary to benign prostatic hyperplasia in large glands (40 to 200 grams) *J Urol* **170**: 1270.

Tan A, Gilling PJG, Kennett K, Fletcher H, Fraundorfer M (2003) Long term results of Holmium laser ablation of the prostate *BJUI* **92**: 707–9.

Tinmouth WW, Habib E, Kim SC, et al. (2005) Change in serum prostate specific antigen concentration after holmium laser enucleation of the prostate: a marker for completeness of adenoma resection? *J Endourol* **19**(5): 550–4.

Westenberg AM, Fraundorfer MR (2006) A randomised trial comparing Holmium laser enucleation versus transurethral resection in the treatment of prostates larger than 40 grams: results at 2 years *Eur Urol* **50**(3): 569–73.

Wilson LC, Gilling PJ, Williams A, Kennett KM, Frampton CM, Gilling PJ, Aho TF, Frampton CM, King CJ, Fraundorfer MR (2008) Holmium laser enucleation of the prostate: results at 6 years *Eur Urol* **53**(4): 744–9.

Chapter 19

Interventional treatment: Thulium laser

Andreas Gross

Key points

- The Thulium:YAG laser is a continuous wave laser for urological soft tissue surgery
- 2 micron wavelength ensures shallow penetration with effective coagulation
- Laser effect is independent from tissue color and vascularization
- Multiple techniques for the treatment of BPO possible.

Being introduced in clinical routine in 2007, the Thulium:YAG 2-micron continuous wave laser (Tm:YAG) is a relatively new tool for the treatment of benign prostatic obstruction. Laser energy is released at a wavelength of 2.013 nm and by this is close to the absorption peak of water. Therefore, laser energy is absorbed by interstitial water, which is ubiquitous in tissue.

Since the Tm:YAG laser is not photoselective, the laser effect is not dependent on tissue coloration. The shallow tissue penetration ensures excellent control of the energy effects and minimizes the risk of collateral damage. Other than the pulsed Ho:YAG laser, being the first choice for the treatment of urinary calculi, the release of laser energy in a continuous wave mode allows more precise incisions with smooth cutting edges. So far, the Tm:YAG laser can be used with a power up to 120 W.

19.1 Technique

Different techniques have been introduced for the Tm:YAG laser prostatectomy. For the energy delivery side-firing as well as front-firing fibres are available. Whereas pure vaporization techniques can be carried out, using either of the fibers, the bare-ended front-firing fiber allows also resection or enculeation of the prostatic adenoma. Energy is delivered into the tissue in a contact mode.

Besides pure vaporization of the tissue mainly two different surgical approaches have been published so far.

- *VapoResection*: Combines vaporization and resection of small TUR-like tissue chips achieving higher tissue ablation than be either technique alone. Using a bare-ended fibre tissue chips are cut from the adenoma by semi-circular movements and pushed into the bladder. At the same time, the vaporization effect at the tip of the fiber is used to increase the amount of removed tissue.

- *VapoEnucleation*: Has been introduced for larger prostate. Instead of cutting out small tissue chips, the prostatic adenoma is removed in as three-lobe technique, consisting out of median lobe and both lateral lobes. The enucleated tissue is morcellated within the bladder. Applying this technique, technically no prostatic size limit occurs. Still the vaporizing effect at the fibre tip, is used to remove adenomous tissue.

19.2 **Functional results**

The Tm:YAG laser has been shown to have effective vaporization capacity in an ex-vivo model (Heinrich et al., 2009). Whereas, vaporization capacity seems to be superior to other vaporizing laser systems, coagulation efficacy remains stable, even with increased power output, again showing superiority to other systems (Bach et al., 2009a, 2009b). However, clinical studies, demonstrating vaporization efficacy in vivo are lacking at this point of time.

Speaking of resection and enucleation techniques, Tm:YAG laser prostatectomy has so far demonstrated effective deobstruction and improvement in QoL and voiding parameter, as well as durability within in intermediate follow-up interval.

One of the main advantages of Tm:YAG laser prostatectomy is the continuus visible laser light, which makes easier handling compared to Ho:YAG laser prostatectomy possible. Because of that, learning enucleation techniques with Tm:YAG is easier.

Complication rate and morbidity is low, transfusion rates are as low as 0.9% in a large cohort study. In a prospective randomized study, Xia et al. may demonstrate the superiority of Tm:YAG prostatectomy over TUR-P with comparable improvement in functional outcome.

Technique	Follow-Up [month]	Patients [n]	Prostate volume [cc]	Total OR-time [min]	Catheter time [d]	Improvement Qmax [ml/s]	IPSS at follow-up [points]
VapoResection (8)	12	54	30.3±4.8	52±21.1	1.7±0.69	15.9	6.9
VapoResection (7)	12	52	59.2±17.7	46.3±16.2	1.90±1.07	15.7	3.5
VapoEnucleation (9)	16.5	62	61.3±24	72±26.6	2.1±1	19.8	6.8
Mixed Techniques (6)	-	208	43.9±23.6	67.7±28.9	2±0.9	15.4	-

Table 19.1

19.3 **Advantages and disadvantages**

The Thulium:YAG 2 micron continuous-wave laser offers multiple treatment options for the treatment of benign prostatic obstruction. Effective deobstruction, even during the initial learning curve as well as durability of the results, with low rates of complication and required re-treatments underline the promising potential of this laser. However, besides being limited to soft tissue surgery, so far long-term follow up, over a period of 18-months, is missing.

- Multiple therapeutic approaches possible (Vaporization, Resection, Enucleation)
- Coagulation efficacy not impaired with increased energy
- All prostate sizes treatable
- Stepwise approach to enucleation possible (from VapoResection to Vapoenuceleation)
- High efficacy with low morbidity.

References

Bach T, Herrmann TRW, Ganzer R, Burchardt M, Gross AJ (2007) RevoLix vaporesection of the prostate: initial results of 54 patients with a 1-year follow-up *World J Urol* **25**: 257–62.

Bach T, Huck N, Wezel F, Haecker A, Gross AJ, Michel MS (2009a) 70 vs. 120 Watt Thulium: YAG 2 micron continuous wave laser for the treatment of benign prostatic hyperplasia. Systematic ex-vivo evaluation *BJU Int* Nov. 13 [Epub ahead of print].

Bach T, Herrmann TRW, Haecker A, Michel MS, Gross AJ (2009b) Thulium:yttrium-aluminum-garnet laser prostatectomy in men with refractory urinary retention *BJU Int* **104**: 361–4.

Bach T, Netsch C, Haecker A, Michel MS, Herrmann TRW, Gross AJ (2009c) Thulium:YAG laser enucleation (VapoEnucleation) of the prostate. Safety and durability during intermediate-term follow-up.

Heinrich E, Wendt-Nordahl G, Honeck P, Alken P, Knoll T, Michel MS, Haecker A (2009) 120 W lithium triborate laser for photoselective vaporization of the prostate: comparison with 80 W potassium-titanyl-phosphat laser in an ex-vivo model *J Endourol* Dec. 3 [Epub ahead of print].

Teichmann HO, Herrmann TR, Bach T (2007) Technical aspects of lasers in urology *World J Urol* **25**: 221–225.

Bach T, Herrmann TRW, Cellarius C, Gross AJ (2007) Bladder neck inzision using a 70 Watt 2 micron continuous wave laser (RevoLix) *World J Urol* **25**: 263–7.

Wendt-Nordahl G, Huckele S, Honeck P, Alken P, Knoll T, Michel MS, Haecker A (2008) Systemic evaluation of a recently introduced 2-micron continuous wave thulium laser for vaporesection of the prostate *J Endourol* **22**: 1041–5.

Xia Sj, Zhuo J, Sun XW, Han BM, Shao Y, Zhang YN (2008) Thulium: YAG laser versus standard transurethral resection of the prostate: A randomized prospective trial *Eur Urol* **53**: 382–90.

Chapter 20

Interventional treatment: Diode laser

Michael Seitz

Key points

- Due to considerable optical penetration depth at 800 to 1100 nm, diode lasers and lasers near the Nd:YAG wavelengths of 1064nm, produce profound tissue coagulation of up to 10 mm, which increases with increased power (W)
- Due to profound tissue coagulation depth at 800–1100 nm diode lasers are not suitable to treat larger prostates since the tissue ablation effect decreases with time and the side effects such as sloughing, incontinence and reoperation rates increase significantly
- At certain wavelengths such as 1300–1500 nm, enucleation and bladder neck incision are feasible with diode lasers
- Current data are inadequate for assessment and for recommendation of diode lasers in the clinical routine. Modulating the pulsing rhythm only seems to be not the suitable option to overcome the wavelength-based disadvantages (deep optical penetration depth).

Diode lasers for the treatment of BPH are available at different wavelenghts. While low power diode lasers at wavelengths between 805 nm and 850 nm were used for interstitial laser coagulation (Pow-Sang et al., 1995; Cromeens et al., 1996; Parapvat et al., 1996; de la Rosette et al., 1997; Daehlin & Hedlund, 1999; Martenson & de la Rosette, 1999), diode lasers emitting light at 940 nm, 980 nm, 1320 nm, and 1470 nm are currently tested for the vaporization of the prostate (Seitz et al., 2007a, b; Seitz et al., 2009a, b, c; Sroka et al., 2007).

In preclinical studies with an ex-vivo autologous blood-perfused porcine kidney model, the diode lasers (≥50 Watt) at 940 nm, 980 nm, and 1470 nm have shown higher tissue ablation capacities in comparison to the KTP laser at 80 Watt and similar hemostasis. However, in contrast to the 80 W KTP-laser, the coagulation zones at 50 Watt differ monumentally. Diode lasers emitting light at 940 nm and 980 nm show in the kidney model a coagulation depth between 8.4 and 9.6 mm indicating a deeper tissue penetration and more profound tissue damage (Seitz et al., 2009a, b, c). With a penetration depth of 3.4 mm the diode laser at 1470 nm seems to be more favourable (KTP ~1.1 mm). It is questionable whether the results from an ex-vivo kidney model reflect the condition in human prostates in every aspect. However, since the specific heat capacities in kidney (3.89 kJ/kg per degree kelvin) and prostate (3.80 kJ/kg per degree kelvin) are almost equivalent, isolated, blood-perfused, porcine kidney seems to be a valuable model, especially for the investigation of laser procedures, in which the heat sink is of the utmost importance (Figure 20.1) (Cooper & Trezek, 1972; Reich et al., 2004).

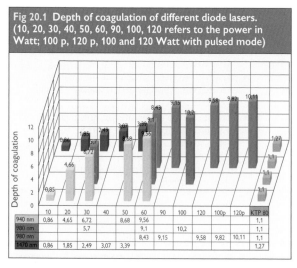

Fig 20.1 Depth of coagulation of different diode lasers.
(10, 20, 30, 40, 50, 60, 90, 100, 120 refers to the power in Watt; 100 p, 120 p, 100 and 120 Watt with pulsed mode)

	10	20	30	40	50	60	90	100	120	100p	120p	KTP 80
940 nm	0,86	4,65	6,72		8,68	9,56						1,1
980 nm			5,7		9,1		10,2					1,1
980 nm						8,43	9,15		9,58	9,82	10,11	1,1
1470 nm	0,86	1,85	2,49	3,07	3,39							1,27

On the other hand, the evaluation in human cadaver prostates showed similar results as in the porcine model. The ablation effect of the diode laser at 980 nm (100–200 W) is two-to-three-times larger than the vaporization zone of the KTP laser (80 W) or the diode laser at 1470 nm (50 W). Also, in human cadaver prostates diode lasers at 980 nm demonstrate a distinct deeper coagulation

(2 to 3.4-times) than the KTP laser device at 80 W or the diode laser at 1470 nm (50 W) (Seitz et al., 2009a). Therefore, the diode laser is able to combine very high tissue ablation properties with the benefit of excellent haemostasis due to deep coagulation.

> However, due to the laser's deep coagulation zones in the 940 nm and 980 nm generators, there may be a hazard of violating underlying structures such as the neurovascular bundles and the external sphincter, which may cause erectile dysfunction and incontinence (Ruszat et al., 2009).

Unfortunately, the value of the human cadaver prostates is limited, since there is no blood perfusion, which is one of the main absorbers at wavelengths between 500 and 1000 nm. Therefore, in vivo studies on canine prostates were carried out to evaluate the diode lasers. At 940 nm the dog prostate tissue was treated with a generator output level of 200 Watt. The mean extension of the coagulation zone was 4.31 mm and the ablation capacity was estimated to be up to 1500 mm³/min (Seitz et al., 2009b). In contrast, the diode laser at 1470 nm produced a coagulation rim of 2.3 mm and the tissue removal ability reached ~400 mm³/min (Seitz et al., 2009c).

Table 20.1

Wavelength	Absorbers	Coagulation	Ablation	Advantage	Disadvantage
~800 nm	Tissue ↑↑↑ Haemoglobin↑↑↑ water↑(↑)	↑↑↑	(↑)	Gooed coagulation and deep tissue penetration for e.g. ILC	No suffivient vaporazation
940 nm	Tissue ↑↑↑ Haemoglobin↑↑↑ water↑↑	↑↑↑	↑↑↑	> 100 W very good vaporization, power up to 300 W possible	deep tissue penetration
980 nm	Tissue ↑↑↑ Haemoglobin↑↑↑ water↑↑	↑↑↑	↑↑↑	> 100 W very good vaporization, power up to 300 W possible	deep tissue penetration
1320 nm	Tissue (↑) water↑↑↑↑	↑↑	↑↑	~90–100 W good vaporization; moderate cutting ability Moderate tissue penetration = good hemostasis	Output power only ~100 Watt
1470 nm	Tissue (↑) water↑↑↑↑	↑↑	↑↑	~90–100W good vaporization; moderate cutting ability Moderate tissue penetration = good hemostasis	Output power only ~100 Watt
532 nm	Tissue ↑↑↑ Haemoglobin↑↑↑↑ Water(↑)	↑	↑↑↑	very good vaporization, small to moderate tissue penetration = good hemostasis, moderate cutting ability	At 80 Watt less effective in comparison to 120 Watt

Currently only a limited number of studies have been investigating the clinical applications of diode laser prostatectomy with a maximum follow-up of 1 year. While all studies show a high intraoperative safety and excellent haemostatic properties, reports on the long-term durability and safety are inconsistent. In a preliminary clinical study on 10 patients, the diode laser at 1470 nm demonstrated an improvement in the IPSS after 12 months from 16.3 to 5.0, and the quality of live score (QoL) fell 3.3 to 0.9. Also Qmax increased from 8.9 ml/s preoperatively to 22.4 ml/s after the operation but reoperation rates were 20% due to laser failure in the treatment of a prominent midlobe [8].

Typically for the majority of available diode laser boxes, the clinical efficacy and safety wasn't proved by clinical studies. In this context advertising and the contineous increase of power up to 300 W plus should be considered with caution.

In a single-centre prospective study comparing a 200 Watt high-power diode laser at 980 nm to a 120 W Greenlight laser ($\lambda = 532$ nm) finally 117 treated patients were treated in both groups. Both laser devices provided rapid tissue ablation; the high power diode laser at 980 nm was more favourable in terms of haemostasis during and after surgery, despite the hemostasis of HPS was excellent. However, higher rates of urinary retention (20%), urgency (24%), urge incontinence (7%), bladder neck strictures (15%), stress incontinence (9%) and tissue necrosis after diode laser ablation of the prostate are indications of deep tissue damage. The authors found high-power diode laser vaporization of the prostate at 980 nm to be in a premature state for treating LUTS secondary to BPH (Ruszat et al., 2009). As one of the most surprising results the researchers found complications which were know years before only with former Nd:YAG lasers: massive tissue necrosis and sloughing up to 6–12 months and a high reoperation rate, postoperatively.

Fig 20.2 2 Necrotic prostatic after high-powered diode laser treatment of the prostate, causing irritative and obstructive voiding disorders months after surgery. N=necrotic prostatic tissue, V=veromontanum, PC=deobstructed, re-epithelized prostatic cavity.

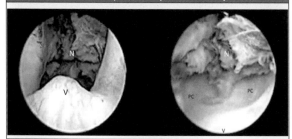

Later, others investigated the diode laser at 980 nm at 100W with 0.1 s pulse length and 0.01 pulse interval in 52 patients and found significant durable improvements in Qmax, post voiding residual urine (PVR) and IPSS-QoL score. In this single-centre and single-surgeon series, no severe complications were reported, including any cases of urinary incontinence, significant irritative symptoms, retrograde ejaculation or worsening of erectile function Ruszat et al., 2009). A subsequent investigation on diode laser vaporization at 980 nm in 47 patients by a Turkish study group revealed a distinct improvement in IPPS and QoL. There was no deterioration in erectile function. The most common postoperative complications were retrograde ejaculation (31.7%) and irritative symptoms (23.4%) (Erol et al., 2009).

In summary, diode laser prostatectomy is feasible. Nevertheless, despite its favourable intraoperative safety, long-term follow-up and large scale trials will be needed to finally evaluate the technique in the future. From the clinical point of view, diode laser vaporization with generators emitting light between 900–1000 nm should be taken with a pinch of salt due to their deep penetration depth since they might lead to damage of underlying structures such as the neurovascular bundle, rectum or external sphincter. On the other hand, diode lasers at 1470 nm have not only a good vaporization ability but also a reasonable and safe tissue penetration depth. This might offer a side-fire operation technique but also a HoLEP-like procedure with a high safety profile.

References

Cooper TE, Trezek GJ (1972) A probe technique for determining the thermal conductivity of tissue *J Heat Transfer* **94**: 133.

Cromeens DM, Johnson DE, Stephens LC, Gray KN (1996) Visual laser ablation of the canine prostate with a diffusing fiber and an 805-nanometer diode laser *Lasers Surg Med* **19**: 135–42.

Daehlin L, Hedlund H (1999) Interstitial laser coagulation in patients with lower urinary tract symptoms from benign prostatic obstruction: treatment under sedoanalgesia with pressure-flow evaluation *BJU Int* **84**: 628–36.

de la Rosette JJ, Muschter R, Lopez MA, Gillatt D (1997) Interstitial laser coagulation in the treatment of benign prostatic hyperplasia using a diode-laser system with temperature feedback *Br J Urol* **80**: 433–8.

Erol A, Cam K, Tekin A, Memik O, Coban S, Ozer Y. High power diode laser vaporization of the prostate: preliminary results for benign prostatic hyperplasia *J Urol* **182**: 1078–82.

Martenson AC, de la Rosette JJ Interstitial laser coagulation in the treatment of benign prostatic hyperplasia using a diode laser system: results of an evolving technology *Prostate Cancer Prostatic Dis* **2**: 148–54.

Pow-Sang M, Orihuela E, Motamedi M, Pow-Sang JE, Cowan DF, Dyer R, Warren MM (1995) Thermocoagulation effect of diode laser radiation in the human prostate: acute and chronic study *Urology* **45**: 790–4.

Prapavat V, Roggan A, Walter J, Beuthan J, Klingbeil U, Muller G. In vitro studies and computer simulations to assess the use of a diode laser (850 nm) for laser-induced thermotherapy (LITT) *Lasers Surg Med* **18**: 22–33.

Reich O, Bachmann A, Schneede P, Zaak D, Sulser T, Hofstetter A (2004) Experimental comparison of high power (80 W) potassium titanyl phosphate laser vaporization and transurethral resection of the prostate *J Urol* **171**: 2502–4.

Ruszat R, Seitz M, Wyler SF, Muller G, Rieken M, Bonkat G, Gasser TC, Reich O, Bachmann A (2009) Prospective single-centre comparison of 120-W diode-pumped solid-state high-intensity system laser vaporization of the prostate and 200-W high-intensive diode-laser ablation of the prostate for treating benign prostatic hyperplasia *BJU Int* **104**: 820–5.

Seitz M, Sroka R, Gratzke C, Schlenker B, Steinbrecher V, Khoder W, Tilki D, Bachmann A, Stief C, Reich O (2007a) The diode laser: a novel side-firing approach for laser vaporisation of the human prostate-immediate efficacy and 1-year follow-up *Eur Urol* **52**: 1717–22.

Seitz M, Ackermann A, Gratzke C, Schlenker B, Ruszat R, Bachmann A, Stief C, Reich O, Sroka R (2007b) Diode laser: Ex vivo studies on vaporization and coagulation characteristics *Urologe A* **46**: 1242–7.

Seitz M, Reich O, Gratzke C, Schlenker B, Karl A, Bader M, Khoder W, Fischer F, Stief C, Sroka R (2009a) High-power diode laser at 980 nm for the treatment of benign prostatic hyperplasia: ex vivo investigations on porcine kidneys and human cadaver prostates *Lasers Med Sci* **24**: 172–8.

Seitz M, Bayer T, Ruszat R, Tilki D, Bachmann A, Gratzke C, Schlenker B, Stief C, Sroka R, Reich O (2009b) Preliminary evaluation of a novel side-fire diode laser emitting light at 940 nm, for the potential treatment of benign prostatic hyperplasia: ex-vivo and in-vivo investigations *BJU Int* **103**: 770–5.

Seitz M, Ruszat R, Bayer T, Tilki D, Bachmann A, Stief C, Sroka R, Reich O (2009c) Ex vivo and in vivo investigations of the novel 1,470 nm diode laser for potential treatment of benign prostatic enlargement *Lasers Med Sci* **24**: 419–24.

Sroka R, Ackermann A, Tilki D, Reich O, Steinbrecher V, Hofstetter A, Stief CG, Seitz M (2007a) In-vitro comparison of the tissue vaporisation capabilities of different lasers *Med Laser Appl* **22**: 227–31.

Chapter 21

Risk-adapted management of BPH

Ingrid Berger and Stephan Madersbacher

Key points

Senior Adults

- Age, co-morbidity, urodynamic considerations and treatment related complications need to be considered
- All drugs currently licensed seem to be safe and effective in the elderly; minimal invasive procedures are an alternative to TURP in patients with high-anaesthesiologic risks.

Patients at risk of progression

- BPH/BPE/BPO are progressive disorders
- prostate volume is the strongest predictor for the risk of acute urinary retention and the need for surgery
- Plant extracts and α-blockers have—in contrast to 5 -reductase inhibitors—no relevant impact on the natural history of the disease
- A risk-stratified management as elaborated herein seems to be advisable.

Prevalences of benign prostatic hyperplasia (BPH), benign prostatic enlargement (BPE), benign prostatic obstruction (BPO) and lower urinary tract symptoms (LUTS) increase almost linearly with age.

Hence it is a disease of the elderly. Demographic changes with a three-fold increase of men older than 85yrs in the next 20yrs and the high-comorbidity in the elderly renders the optimal management of senior adults with this disease a relevant and important issue.

Several population-based cross-sectional and longitudinal studies and the placebo-arms of long-term medical trials have provided strong evidence for the progressive nature of BPH:

- The Olmsted County study has shown that 31% of men have at least a three-point increase in the AUA-symptom index over the 92-month study period
- The longitudinal Veterans Affairs study demonstrated that 36% of patients with BPH assigned to watchful waiting required invasive therapy within 5 years. The risk of acute urinary retention has been estimated as 23% for an average 60-year old man if he survived fur-ther 20 years.

In the 7th decade of life, BPH is present in more than 60%, BPE in around of 40% and LUTS in 30–40%.

Geriatric patients are not specifically age defined, "Most patients will be over 65 years of age but the problems best dealt with by the speciality of Geriatric Medicine become much more common in the 80+ age group".

There is a close correlation between the degree of co-morbidity and life-expectancy.

Within the past decade, several risk factors for disease progression have been identified, the clinical most relevant being prostate volume. This has led to a risk-stratified approach.

21.1 **Management of elderly patients ("senior adults")**

21.1.1 Comorbidity – life expectancy

There exists no generally accepted definition of a "senior adult". Should this definition be based on chronological age and if, which cut-off should be used? Which role does the degree of co-morbidity play and how should it be quantified? The European definition of Geriatric Medicine officially approved by the Geriatric Medicine Section of the UEMS (Union Europénne des Médécins Spécialistes) at its meeting in Malta in May 2008 (UEMS—GMS, Malta, May 3rd, 2008) describes geriatric patients as having "a high degree of frailty and multiple pathologies, requiring a holistic approach". Geriatric Medicine therefore has to "exceed organ orientated medicine offering additional therapy in a multidisciplinary team setting, the main aim of which is to optimise the functional status of the older person and improve the quality of life and autonomy".

21.1.2 Urodynamic considerations

The ageing lower urinary tract is characterized by a number of age-related urodynamic changes, such as a decline of maximum flow rate (Qmax), voided volume, bladder capacity, bladder compliance paralleled by an increase of post-void residual volume, bladder outflow obstruction and the incidence of detrusor overactivity. The pathomechanisms leading to these changes are multiple and involve BPO, age-related structural changes of urinary bladder, central nervous system changes with impaired bladder control and fluid imbalances (e.g. nocturnal polyuria, renal/cardiovascular alterations). These diverse mechanisms indicate that the prostate, i.e. BPO is not the only factor attributing to the development of LUTS in the elderly.

> Less than 30% of patients older than 80yrs are urodynamically obstructed when they present with a Qmax of 10–15ml/sec.

This underlines the declining role of BPO in the pathogenesis of LUTS in the elderly and emphasises the role of a through assessment (including urodynamics in selected cases) particularly prior prostatectomy.

21.1.3 Treatment options in senior adults

Several factors need to be considered when choosing a treatment strategy:

- Age
- Individual anesthesiologic risk and comorbidity
- Degree of BPO
- Prostate size and shape (e.g. middle lobe)
- Treatment related complications
- Risk of disease progression
- Presence of an indwelling catheter
- Neurologic disorders as well as the efficacy
- Costs of treatment modalities.

21.1.4 Medical therapy

The aim of medical therapy in senior adults is not different to that of younger men, i.e. to control/improve symptoms and quality of life and/or to prevent long-term complications such as acute urinary retention or BPH-related surgery. Current knowledge suggests that treatment efficacy of medical therapy is comparable in younger men and senior adults. However many clinical trials have excluded geriatric patients. Specific factors that need to be considered in senior adults are the issue of polypharmacy and altered drug metabolism. With aging, physiological changes raise drugs levels in serum and cerebrospinal fluid thus increasing the odds of adverse events (e.g. neurological side effects of some anticholinergics).

As biological and chronological age have no relevant impact on indication and efficacy of medical therapy, the reader is referred to the respective chapters in this book. We therefore concentrate herein on side effects.

- **plant extracts:** the major advantage of plant extracts is the lack of side effects; the down-side is that the efficacy is not convincingly demonstrated; therefore plant extracts are not recommended by BPH-guidelines

- **α_1-blockers:** the main difference between α-blockers is related to the rate of side effects. In general, alfuzosin (in particular, the 10mg once daily formulation) and tamsulosin are better tolerated than terazosin and doxazosin in terms of vasodilatory adverse events. Tamsulosin has no relevant interaction with several antihypertensive agents and has been specifically tested in senior adults.

- **5α-reductase inhibitors**: the only relevant side-effects of 5ARIs relate to sexuality, i.e. loss of libido, erectile dysfunction, reduced ejaculate volume and gynaecomastia. As these side effects are rare and of—usually—little relevance for senior adults, 5ARIs are considered safe in this group of patients.

- **anticholinergics:** the high prevalence of detrusor overactivity in elderly men and recent data suggesting that a combination of anticholinergics and α-blockers is safe in men with LUTS renders this approach attractive. Particularly in senior adults anticholinergics that pass the blood-brain barrier (oxybutinin and tolterodine) can lead to serious CNS side effects. Trospium chloride that does not pass the (healthy) blood-brain barrier and M3-selective anticholinergics (darifenacin/solifenacin) are considered safe with this respect and are therefore preferable in senior adults.

21.1.5 Surgery and minimal invasive therapy

Monopolar TURP is considered the gold-standard therapy, yet treatment related morbidity is an issue, particularly in senior adults. Side effects include bleeding, dilution hyponatraemia (including TUR-syndrome), incontinence and stricture formation. The advent of bipolar TUR has abandoned the risk of the TUR-syndrome. Elderly patients with large prostates and pace makers should be treated with bipolar TURP; neoadjuvant use of 5ARIs is indicated in men with significant BPE to reduce the risk of bleeding.

Risk of bleeding and anaesthetic requirements for TURP are the driving forces behind the development of minimal invasive procedures and three procedures (transurethral microwave thermotherapy TUMT; transurethral needle ablation TUNA and laser prostatectomy) gained wide-spread acceptance.

Only TUMT and TUNA can be performed under local anaesthesia, both procedures have been proven to be safe and effective, although improvements of symptoms and particularly of objective parameters are less than after TURP and retreatment rates considerable higher. Nevertheless TUMT and TUNA are established procedures particularly for those with high anaesthetic risk or unfit for surgery.

Intraprostatic Botulinum toxin A injection is currently studied as a minimally invasive alternative; as this procedure can also be performed under local anaesthesia, it is attractive for elderly, frail patients with high anaesthetic risks.

Two laser techniques, i.e. transurethral holmium laser enucleation of the prostate (HoLEP) and photoselective prostatic vaporization by green light at a wave length of 532 nm (KTP) have gained acceptance. Both procedures, however, require general anaesthesia, such as conventional TURP or open prostatectomy. The major advantage to bipolar TURP is the minimal risk of bleeding; particularly KTP-laser vaporisation. This procedure can be safely performed even under ongoing anticoagulant therapy, an important aspect for geriatric patients with bleeding disorders or under anticoagulant therapy.

21.2 **Management of patients at high risk of disease progression**

21.2.1 **Who is at risk?**

In this chapter disease progression is defined as acute urinary retention or the need for surgery (and not by worsening of symptoms). MTOPS was the first long-term medical trial that applied the concept of disease progression. Over 4.5 years approx. 20% of patients in the placebo-arm developed a disease progression defined by:

- A rise of the AUA-symptom index by >4
- Development of acute urinary retention (AUR)
- BPO-related renal insufficiency and
- BPO-related urinary incontinence and
- BPO-related recurrent urinary tract infection.

The by far most frequent event leading to disease progression was a rise in the AUA-score in 78% followed by AUR in 12%. AUR resulted in prostatectomy in the vast majority of patients.

Prostate volume and—as a proxy parameter—PSA are associated with symptom deterioration but also with progression to AUR and the need for surgery. Although the absolute risk of disease progression can vary substantially among individuals, men with a prostate volume >30 ml have a 3 times higher risk for AUR and a significantly greater risk of requiring BPH-related surgery. Analyses of the placebo-arms of long-term medical trials also demonstrated a close correlation between prostate volume and the risk of AUR: over 4yrs 8% of men with prostate volumes 14–41ml, 12% with prostate volumes 42–57ml and 21% of those with prostate volumes >58ml developed AUR. Apart from prostate volume, Qmax, age and the degree of LUTS have been shown to be correlated to the risk of AUR and surgery.

21.2.2 Medical therapy

21.2.2.1 Plant extracts

To date only 5 trials meeting WHO-BPH criteria (12 months study duration, randomised against placebo or standard therapy) have been reported for plant extracts. In none of these trials changes for prostate volume or PSA have been demonstrated, data on the impact on the risk of AUR of surgery are not available. Based on the current data, plant extracts are not capable of altering the natural history of the disease and are therefore not indicated in patients with a high risk of disease progression.

21.2.2.2 α-blockers

Although other mechanism of action might exist, α-blockers inhibit 1-adrenoreceptor mediated sympathetic stimulation and relax smooth muscle tone in the prostate and bladder neck. In situ analysis of tissue taken from patients treated with terazosin/ doxazosin suggested that these agents induce apoptosis in the prostatic glandular epithelium and stroma. However, large scale, long-term trials failed to demonstrate any effect of α-blockers on prostate volume. MTOPS showed that patients on doxazosin had an identical increase of prostate volume (+24% over 4.5yrs) than under placebo. Consistent with these findings, treatment with α-blockers has not been shown to reduce the long-term risk of AUR and BPH-related surgery. In the MTOPS-trial, doxazosin delayed the time to AUR for about two years yet did not significantly reduce the cumulative incidence at four years compared to placebo. Similarly, in the ALTESS study, alfuzosin did not reduce the risk of AUR compared to placebo. Although there was a trend towards lower incidence of BPH-related surgery in the alfuzosin group, this trend did not reach statistical significance.

21.2.2.3 5α-reductase inhibitors

There exists considerable evidence to support the view that 5ARIs reduce the risk of AUR and the need for surgery. This risk reduction is mediated via the effect of 5ARIs on prostate volume by inhibiting 5-reductase type II (finasteride) or types I and II (dutasteride). Prolonged administration of 5ARIs leads to a prostate volume reduction by 20–30%. For both 5ARIs currently in clinical use (finasteride/dutasteride) long-term placebo-controlled trials have shown that 5ARIs capable to reduce the risk of AUR or BPH-related surgery by approximately 50%. This evidence is based in three long term trials with finasteride (PROWESS, PLESS, MTOPS) and the three 2-yrs placebo-controlled trials with dutasteride.

21.2.2.4 *Combination therapy*

Given the distinct modes of action of 5ARIs and α-blockers and resultant differences in therapeutic benefit, the rationale for using combined therapy is clear: rapid symptom relief by α-blockers and long-term risk reduction by 5ARIs. The superiority of combination therapy on LUTS and a composite progression definition had been convincingly documented in MTOPS and the 2 years data of the CombAT-trial (dustasteride vs. tamsulosin vs. combination). The MTOPS trial, however, has shown that combination therapy (finasteride plus doxazosin) is not significantly superior to finasteride monotherapy regarding the risk of AUR and the need for surgery. The CombAT-trial was designed to specifically recruit patients at high risk of disease progression based on prostate volume. The mean baseline volume in CombAT (53 ml) was substantially higher than e.g. in MTOPS (36ml). At the 4-years study end data on AUR and need for surgery will be generated. This landmark study will provide new insights on the role of combination therapy in patients at high risk of disease progression.

The combination of α-blocker and anticholinergic has not been tested regarding its potential impact on the natural history. Given their mode of action it is unlikely that this approach will have an effect with this respect.

21.2.3 **Risk-stratified management**

A more thorough understanding of the natural history of the disease, the identification of risk factors for disease progression and the availability of drugs capable to alter the natural history led to the concept of a risk-stratified management (Figure 21.1).

Patients are primarily stratified based on symptom status. Those with mild symptoms are best managed by watchful waiting, the "prophylactic" use of 5ARIs in asymptomatic men with larger prostates is scientifically sound yet currently not recommended mainly for socioeconomic reasons. Patients with moderate/severe LUTS and low risk of progression (i.e. prostate volumes <30–40 ml) should be treated by α-blockers. Those at a higher risk of disease progression should receive combination therapy; the duration of combination therapy (i.e. when to stop the α-blocker) is still a matter

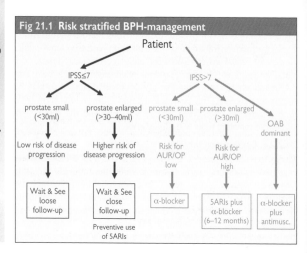

Fig 21.1 Risk stratified BPH-management

of debate. According to one trial, the α-blocker can be safely omitted after 6–9 months in the majority of patients. In patients with a dominance of storage symptoms and no relevant BPO a combination of anticholinergics and α_1-blocker is advisable.

In 2009, management of senior adults with LUTS is based on symptom status, quality of life impairment, risk of disease progression, chronological and biological age, co-morbidity and polypharmacy. All medical therapies currently on the market are safe and effective in senior adults, particular caution is necessary with the use of anticholinergics. In the presence of a strong/absolute indication for surgery, TURP is still unsurpassed regarding clinical efficacy. In patients with high anesthesiologic risks, procedures avoiding general anaesthesia such as TUMT and TUNA are preferable, laser procedures for those with bleeding disorders.

A thorough understanding of the natural history of the disease, the identification of risk factors for disease progression and the availability of drugs capable to alter the natural history led to the concept of a risk-stratified management as elaborated above.

Medical therapy should not be prolonged uncritically. If lower urinary tract function deteriorates, desobstructive minimal invasive or conventional surgery should be initiated to avoid irreversible detrusor failure. In sa called high-risk patients preferably laser or bipolare surgery should be used.

References

Chapple CR, Wein AJ, Abrams P et al. (2008) Lower urinary tract symptoms revisited: a broader clinical perspective *Eur Urol* **54**: 563–69.

Donohue JF, Sharma H, Abraham R, Natalwala S, Thomas DR, Foster MC (2002) Transurethral prostate resection and bleeding: a randomized, placebo controlled trial of role of finasteride for decreasing operative blood loss *J Urol* **168**: 2024–6.

Emberton M, Zinner N, Michel MC et al. (2007) Managing the progression of lower urinary tract symptoms/benign prostatic hyperplasia: therapeutic options for the man at risk *BJU Int* **100**: 249–53.

Madersbacher S, Alivizatos G, Nordling J et al. (2004) EAU 2004 guidelines on assessment, therapy, and follow-up of men with lower urinary tract symptoms suggestive of benign prostatic obstruction (BPH guidelines) *Eur Urol* **46**: 547–54.

Madersbacher S, Marszalek M, Lackner J et al. (2007) The long-term outcome of medical therapy for BPH *Eur Urol* **51**: 1522–33.

Madersbacher S, Berger I, Ponholzer A et al. (2008) Plant extracts: sense or nonsene? *Curr Opin Urol* **18**: 16–20.

Marszalek M, Ponholzer A, Pusman M et al. (2009) Transurethral resection of the prostate *Eur Urol Update Series* **8**: 504–12.

McConnell JD, Roehrborn CG, Bautista OM et al. (2003) The long-term effect of doxazosin, finasteride, and combination therapy on the clinical progression of benign prostatic hyperplasia *N Engl J Med* **349**: 2387–98.

Naspro R, Bachmann A, Gilling P et al (2009) A review of the recent evidence (2006-2008) for 532-nm photoselective laser vaporisation and holmium laser enucleation of the prostate *Eur Urol* **55**: 1345–57.

Roehrborn CG, Siami P, Barkin J et al. (2008) The effects of dutasteride, tamsulosin and combination therapy on lower urinary tract symptoms in men with benign prostatic hyperplasia and prostatic enlargement: 2-year results from the CombAT study *J Urol* **179**: 616–21.

Ruszat R, Wyler S, Foster T et al. (2007) Safety and effectiveness of photoselective vaporization of the prostate (PVP) in patients on ongoing anticoagulation *Eur Urol* **51**: 1031–8.

Chapter 22

Complications of BPH

Jens J. Rassweiler

Key points

- Benign prostatic hyperplasia is associated with significant side effects
- There is a need to evaluate these side effects as a basis for treatment decision
- Interventional management of benign prostatic hyperplasia is also associated with complications. Such side-effects may occur peri- as well as postoperatively
- Recent technological improvement of the different treatment techniques (ie TURP, laserablation, laserenucleation) has resulted in a significant decrease of perioperative complication rate.

Despite the introduction of alternative techniques, transurethral resection of the prostate (TURP) still represents the reference standard in the operative management of benign prostatic hyperplasia. TURP underwent significant technical improvement during the last decade with major impact on the incidence of intra- and postoperative complications (Tables 22.1, 22.2). Additionally, prevention and management of complications based on long-term experience is presented discussing the impact of further technological improvement.

Table 22.1 Incidence and type of intra- and perioperative complications after TURP

Type of complication	Mebust 1989	Doll 1992	Haupt 1997	Borboroglu 1999	Kuntz 2004	Reich 2008
Technical complication (%)						
Clot retention	3.3	11.0	1.9	1.3	5.0	n.a.
Bleeding & Transfusion	6.4	22.0	2.2	0.4	2.0	2.9
TUR-syndrome	2.0	n.a.	0.3	0.8	0.0	1.4
Capsular perforation	0.9	10.0	n.a.	n.a.	4.0	n.a.
Hydronephrosis	0.3	n.a.	0.0	0.0	0.0	n.a.
Epididymitis/UTI	3.9	25.0	1.6	4.0	4.0	3.6
Urosepsis	0.2	3.0	0.2	0.0	0.0	n.a.
Failure to void	6.5	3.0	n.a.	7.1	5.0	5.8
Incontinence	n.a.	38.0	0.3	n.a.	1.0	n.a.
Associated morbidity (%)						
Cardiac arrhythmia	1.1	n.a.	0.4	1.3	n.a.	n.a.
Myocardial infarction	0.05	0.5	0.2	0.2	0.0	n.a.
Pulmonary embolism	n.a.	n.a.	0.1	n.a.	0.0	n.a.
COPD	0.5	n.a.	0.1	n.a.	n.a.	n.a.
Mortality	0.23	0.8	0.1	0.0	0.0	0.1

n.a. = not available

22.1 Indications and contraindications for TURP

Basically the following facts represent the complications of conservative management of BPH, such as:

- Recurrent urinary tract infection due to bladder outlet obstruction
- Recurrent episodes of urinary retention
- Presence of bladder calculi
- Recurrent hematuria due to bladder outlet obstruction
- Renal insufficiency due to BPH.

Table 22.2 Perioperative complications after TURP—comparison of two decades

Authors	N	Transfusion (%)	Revision (%)	Infection (%)	TUR–syndrome
Mebust 1989	3885	6.4	n.a.	2.3	2.0
Doll 1992	388	22.0	3.0.	14.0	n.a.
Horninger 1996	1211	7.6	n.a.	n.a.	2.8
Haupt 1997	934	2.2	n.a.	n.a.	0.3
Zwergel 1998	214	14.6	n.a.	n.a.	0.8
Borboroglu 1999	520	0.4	n.a.	2.1	0.8
Kuntz 2004	100	2.0	3.0	4.0	0.0
Muzzonigro 2004	113	7.1	n.a.	n.a.	0.0
Berger 2004[+]	271	2.6	n.a.	n.a.	1.1
Rassweiler 2006	7707	3.0	5.0	3.5	0.8
Reich 2008	10654	2.9	5.6	3.6	1.4

n.a. = not available, [+]with coagulating intermittent cutting

Contraindications represent untreated urinary infection and coagulation disorders. High-risk patients have to be checked carefully by the cardiologist or anesthesiologist to minimize the risk of associated morbidity (Table 22.1).

22.2 **Resection techniques**

Different systematic approaches for TURP have been proposed:, Nesbit described a procedure starting with the ventral parts of the gland (i.e. between 11 and 1 o'clock) followed by both lateral lobes, the mid-lobe, and finishing with the apex, whereas Flocks preferred to start with the mid-lobe followed by the lateral lobes being segmented at 9 and 3 o'clock. In Germany, the technique developed by Mauermayer and Hartung gained popularity. TURP is divided in fours steps: mid-lobe resection, paracollicular TUR, resection of lateral lobes and ventral parts, and apical resection.

Further development included:

• The use of suprapubic trocar system,
• The introduction of continuous-flow resectoscopes
• And the introduction of video-assisted resection.

22.3 **TURP technology**

Not cursive *electroresection* is performed by monopolar, high-frequency current with maximum power for cutting up to 200 W. A microprocessor controlled electrical unit with an active electrode transducing permanently signals to the processor allows real-time adjustment of the power. Since coagulation depth during cutting depends on the intensity of the light bow (i.e. the voltage), the degree of coagulation is adjusted to the individual tissue properties.

Coagulating intermittent cutting was developed to realize blood-sparing TURP by modification of a standard high frequency generator: phases with predominant cutting effect alternate with coagulating phases of constant pulses under control of pulse intervals. Other instrumental alternatives to decrease TURP-morbidity included modified shapes of the electrode (i.e. thick loop), generator modifications enabling vaporization of tissue or additional mechanical ablative effects (i.e. Rotoresect).

Recently, manufacturers (i.e. Gyrus, Vista-ACMI, Olympus, Karl Storz) introduced bipolar devices differing with respect to the shape of the loop and technical solution of *bipolar TURP* (i.e. active and return electrode). High frequency energy (up to 160 W) passes through the conductive irrigation solution (0.9% sodium chloride) resulting to a vapour layer (plasma) containing energy charged particles, which induce tissue disintegration through molecular dissociation. Compared to conventional monopolar systems this leads to lower resection temperature, so that theoretically thermal damage to surrounding tissue is reduced. The use of physiological sodium chloride for irrigation eliminates the risk of TUR-syndrome.

22.4 **Laser prostatectomy**

Alternative ablative technologies include Holmium-YAG laser resection or ablation, and KTP-laser photoselective vaporization of the prostate. These techniques are reported to be virtually bloodless providing short catheter times with comparable functional outcome like TURP see Chapter 16.

22.5 **Intra-operative complications**

Mostly, they are related to the technical difficulties of the procedure including bleeding requiring transfusion and/or postoperative interventions, the TUR-syndrome, and extraperitoneal extravasation due to injury of the prostatic capsule and/or the bladder neck (Tables 22.1, 22.2).

22.5.1 **Bleeding**

Intraoperative haemorrhage occurs due to arterial and venous bleeders. Arterial bleeding can be more pronounced in case of preoperative infection or urinary retention due a congestive prostatic disease. Antiandrogen pre-treatment with finasteride or flutamide may reduce the bleeding tendency. Venous bleeding occurs predominantly due to capsular perforation with opening of venous sinusoids. The amount of intraoperative bleeding also may depend on the size of the gland respectively the resection weight (transfusion rate 9.6 % if gland >60 ml; Reich et al., 2008).

22.5.2 **Technical aspects**

According to the different resection techniques, vascular control of prostatic vessels differs. Whereas in the Mauermeyer-approach the vessels at 5 and 7 o'clock are controlled early, the Nesbit-technique aims to reach first the capsule at the 11 and 1 o'clock position. According to our experience both approaches are comparable and depend on surgeon's preference, only.

Technical improvement of monopolar HF-generators (i.e. microprocessor controlled high-cut, coagulating intermittent cutting) as well as concerning the instrumentarium (i.e. continuous flow resectoscopes, suprapubic trocar systems) resulted in a significant decrease o transfusion rates. Whereas in the eighties transfusion rates of up to 25% have been reported, the incidence has come down to 0.4 to 7.1 %, depending on prostate size and surgeon experience (Table 22.2).

The improved training of TUR using the video technology allows the trainee as well as the mentor to observe every technical step of the procedure comfortably, compared to the cumbersome angulated side-lens-occulars. Since, the amount of bleeding also depends on the resection time, faster resection techniques could contribute to the success.

22.5.3 **Management**

During resection, the following problems with arterial bleeders may occur:

- Arterial flow is directed to the optic
- Bleeding covered by a coagulum or behind prostatic tissue

- Bleeding close to the apex (i.e. 12 o'clock position)
- Bleeding at the bladder neck.

In case of larger arteries, the resectoscope might be used to compress the bleeding (Figure 22.1). After that, the optimal angle visualizing the bleeding stump must be found avoiding any arterial flow directed to the optic. Bleeding arteries have to be coagulated circumferentially, once the resection has reached the capsule, thereby achieving a sealing effect of the stump. Simultaneous recto-digital manipulation might be useful to expose such vessels. Towards the end of resection, careful hemostasis must be performed using

Fig 22.1 Management of arterial bleeds

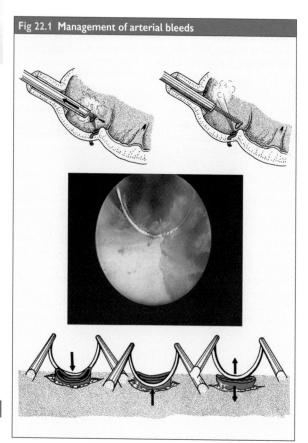

minimal irrigation flow visualizing the source of small arterial bleeders. In particular, bleeders at the bladder neck or apex can be overseen.

Venous bleeders may not be visible during resection and thus cause influx of irrigation fluid. However, if emptying the bladder, the fluid shows significant dark red colour. Venous sinusoids can be coagulated, but in case of associated capsular perforation, this has to be performed with care not to aggravate the perforation. Smaller veins can be occluded by use of the three-way-balloon catheter at the end of the TUR (Figure 22.2).

22.5.4 **Balloon-compression**

The catheter should be blocked with only 20 cc in the prostatic fossa, however, in critical cases, the balloon can be blocked in the bladder (i.e. 60–80 cc) and put under traction to compress the fossa. This can be accomplished by using a gauze knotted around the catheter at the meatus. Blockade of the balloon in the fossa to tamponade smaller veins may remove thrombi of coagulated vessels or lead to rupture of the capsule. Additional recto-digital control with compression of bleeding sources (i.e. 5–10 minutes) may be useful.

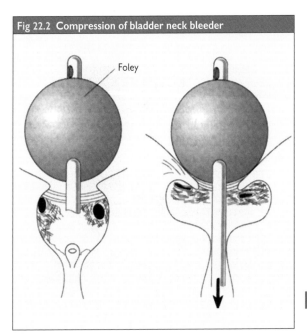

Fig 22.2 Compression of bladder neck bleeder

Foley

22.5.5 **Re-coagulation**

Latest in the recovery room, the irrigation fluid should clear up, otherwise immediate transurethral reintervention with evacuation of tamponade and coagulation of the bleeding site is mandatory to minimize the risk of further complications (i.e. blood transfusion, infection). Bleeding during resection can be reduced by use of alternative energy sources, such as Holmium-laser.

22.5.6 **TUR-syndrome**

The TUR-syndrome is caused by dilulational hyponatremia (serum sodium < 125 mEq/l) due to perforation of capsular veins or sinuses at an early stage of the resection with consecutive absorption/influx of irrigating fluid. It is characterized:

- By mental confusion
- Nausea
- Vomiting
- Hypertension
- Bradycardia
- And/or visual disturbances (if the patient has spinal anesthesia).

Patients under spinal anesthesia may show unrest and cerebral disturbance or shivering as early signs of the TUR-syndrome. Untreated, it may have severe consequences like cerebral and/or pulmonary edema. However, the incidence has significant decreased during the last decades from 3% to less than 1% (Table 22.2).

22.5.6.1 *Diagnosis*

In any suspicion of a TUR-syndrome, immediate check of serum sodium must be performed. Addition of aethylalcohol to the irrigant may allow early detection of influx by analysis of the alcohol content in the exsufflated air. However, because of the low incidence of TUR-syndrome, we do not recommend this routinely.

22.5.6.2 *Management*

Some authors recommend the application of 20 mg furosemide at the end of the resection. For larger glands (>60 cc) the use of a suprapubic trocar is mandatory. Beside the prevention of high-pressure situations during TURP, this manoeuvre optimizes intra-operative visibility dramatically. The Nesbit technique is associated by a higher risk of influx because the capsule is reached at an early stage of the resection.

In any suspicion of a TUR-syndrome, immediate check of serum sodium has to be performed. In case of significant hyponatriemia (i.e. >125 mval/ml), the procedure has to be stopped. Addition of ethylalcohol to the irrigant may allow early detection of influx by analysis of the alcohol content in the exhaled air. However, because of the low incidence, we do not recommend the routinely.

22.5.6.3 *Prevention*

The low indicence of TUR-syndrome is mainly related to the use of low-pressure systems either using the Iglesias-continuous flow resectoscope or more frequently a suprapubic trocar.

However, a dramatic undetected fluid uptake causing cardio-pulmonal problems is possible due to the longer feasible OR time.

> The use of bipolar or laser technology completely avoids the TUR-syndrome, because sodium chloride (0.9%) is used.

22.5.7 **Extravasation**

When the prostatic capsule is injured or the bladder neck is divided, the extravasation of the irrigation fluid is extra-/retroperitoneal in most instances. However, irrigation fluid can also be found intraperitoneally (i.e. by diffusion of large amounts, bladder injury).

22.5.7.1 *Diagnosis*

Palpation and Ultrasound: If the input of irrigation does not correlate with the output together with a palpable increase of abdominal pressure, ultrasound examination has to be performed immediately, to identify intra or retroperitoneal extravasation. Usually, this is associated with complications, such as abdominal pain respiratory insufficiency, and requires drainage.

22.5.7.2 *Management and prevention*

In case of extraperitoneal extravasation, forced diuresis (i.e. 20–40 mg furosemide) may be sufficient. Intraperitoneal fluid collection can be drained percutaneously by insertion of a cystostomy or nephrostomy stent under ultrasonic guidance.

In the case of sodium chloride as irrigiant, the extravasation induces less symptoms and only in case of massive transperitoneal effusion, percutaneous drainage is necessary. If a capsular perforation has been recognized, the irrigation pressure should be reduced (lower the height of the irrigation bag). Evacuation of chips should be performed very carefully, so asnot to increase the perforation (i.e. at bladder neck).

22.5.8 **Injury of orifices**

Such a lesion may occur during resection of large mid-lobes, where primary identification of the ureteral orifices is difficult. Like in TUR of bladder tumours, the management depends on the lesion.

22.5.8.1 *Management and prevention*

In the case of severe ureteral injury a DJ-stent may be indicated, otherwise, sonographic follow-up is sufficient. The stent should be kept indwelling for 2–3 weeks. Identification of the orifices should be mandatory before starting TURP. If this is not possible (i.e. large mid-lobe), care should be taken particularly close to the bladder neck. Suprapubic cystoscopy can be helpful in this situation.

22.5.9 Injury of external sphincter

Not all forms of postoperative incontinence are caused by iatrogenic trauma of the external sphincter muscle. The lesion occurs mainly ventrally (at 12 o'clock), where the veru montanum is not visible as anatomical landmark. Also, if the veru montanum has been resected eventually, there is an increased risk of sphincteric injury. The exact localization of the external sphincter should be checked repeatedly, particularly during apical paracollicular resection.

22.5.9.1 *Prevention*

The localization of the veru montanum should be checked exactly at the beginning of TURP, particularly in cases with large lobes, where the veru might be flattened. Rectal palpation might be helpful to identify the area of external sphincter. If there is a suspicious lesion at the external sphincter, traction at the balloon-catheter should be minimized.

22.6 Postoperative complications

This includes early and late complications such as urethral strictures, which need a certain time to develop.

22.6.1 Bladder tamponade

Recurrent or persisting bleeding usually results in formation of clots and a bladder tamponade requiring evacuation or even re-intervention under anaesthesia (2–5%). Arterial bleeders usually can be identified by a change of clear and red colour of the irrigation outflow (cloudy red spots), whereas venous bleeders result in a dark red continuous irrigation fluid.

22.6.2 Management

Primarily, evacuation of obstructing clots should be performed followed by replacement of the balloon catheter, eventually under rectal palpation. The balloon can be either blocked in the fossa or inflated in the bladder (20–40 cc more than the resection weight) and put under traction. However, this technique does not work in case of active arterial bleeders, particularly at the bladder neck.

Occasionally, due to associated coagulation disorders (i.e. undetected preoperatively), coagulation alone may be insufficient. In such situations, additional recto-digital palpation can be successful to stop the bleeding. Another alternative represents transfemoral superselective embolization.

22.6.3 Infection

The rate of infection is low (i.e. in Baden-Württemberg 3.5 %, Bavaria 2.7 %), however, in the French multicentre study the incidence of post-TURP infection was 21.6 %, including 2.3 % of septic shock. Risk factors of infection include:

- Preoperative bacturia
- Longer duration of the procedure (i.e. >70 min.)
- Preoperative stay >2 days
- Discontinuation of catheter drainage (i.e. evacuation of tamponade).

We recommend a peri-operative antibiotic prophylaxis (i.e. co-trimoxazole, gyrase-inhibitors) as long as the catheter is in place. Concerning postoperative epididydimitis, we also see a low incidence and do not recommend a routine vasectomy simultaneous to TURP.

22.6.4 Urinary retention

Urinary retention (3–9%) is mainly attributed to primary detrusor failure rather than to incomplete resection. Therefore, we are very conservative concerning early repeated TURP in the case of persisting residual urine or micturation problems. Unless TRUS does show any left significant tissue (i.e. ventile effects) the healing of the prostatic fossa should be awaited. Symptomatic treatment can include anti-inflammatory drugs like diclofenac. Especially in the case of decompensation of the detrusor muscle, residual urine may persist above 100 cc for a significant amount of time without presenting a problem to the patient.

22.6.5 Incontinence

Early incontinence may occur frequently (up to 30–40%), however, late iatrogenic stress-incontinence has become a rare event (<0.5%).

22.6.5.1 *Early management*

Early incontinence predominantly is related to urge-symptomatic because of either irritative symptoms (i.e. healing of fossa, associated UTI) or detrusor hyperactivity due to long-lasting BPH. Symptomatic treatment should include time-limited anti-cholinergic selective drugs (tolterodine, darifenacin) as well as anti-inflammatory regimens (i.e. diclofenac).

22.6.5.2 *Urodynamic evaluation*

Persisting (i.e. >6 months) incontinence requires complete investigation including, ascending urethrogram, cystourethroscopy, and urodynamic evaluation. There are several causes for incontinence:

- Sphincter incompetence (30%)
- Detrusor instability (20%)
- Mixed incontinence (30%)
- Residual adenoma (5%)
- Bladder neck contracture (5%)
- urethral stricture (5%).

22.6.5.3 *Late management*

Depending on endoscopic and urodynamic findings, conservative treatment with pelvic floor exercise (combined with TRUS-biofeedback), and electrostimulation might be indicated. Promising experiences with the use of duloxetine (40 mg b.i.d.) must be balanced against the side-effects leading to discontinuation by the patient. Since periurethral injection therapy was not very successful, an artificial sphincter might be indicated for few patients. Recently, higher success rates (67% dry, 92% improvement) were reported by use of inflatable paraurethral balloons and male suburethral sling-systems (ie. Advance, AMS).

22.6.6 **Urethral stricture**

The rate of urethral stricture varies significantly in the literature from 2.2 to 9.8% (Table 22.3). There are two main reasons and localizations: Strictures at the meatus mainly occur due to a false relationship between the size of the instrument (Ch 24–27) and the diameter of the urethral meatus. Bulbar strictures occur due to leakage of monopolar current incase of insufficient isolation by the jelly (i.e. Endosgel).

22.6.6.1 *Prevention*

The jelly should be applied with care in the urethra and along the shaft of the resectoscope. In case of longer resection time, re-application of the jelly is mandatory. Moreover, high cutting current should be avoided. In case of relative meatal or urethral strictures, internal urethrotomy should be performed prior to TURP.

22.6.7 **Bladder neck stenosis**

Bladder neck stenosis (0.3–9.2 %) usually occurs following treatment of smaller glands (i.e. less than 30 g). Therefore, the indication for TURP in case of smaller glands should be taken very carefully. Prophylactic bladder neck incision at the end of the procedure may reduce the incidence. Again, theoretically with the use of bipolar technology, less bladder neck strictures should occur.

22.6.8 **Retrograde ejaculation**

According to the nature of the procedure, retrograde ejaculation occurs in a majority of patients (50–95%). Retrograde ejaculation might be avoided, if the tissue around the veru montaneum (i.e. the

Authors	N	Incontinence (%)	Re-TUR (%)	Impotence (%)	Stricture (%)
Zwergel 1979	232	11.4	n.a.	n.a.	4.4
Doll 1992	388	9.0	1.5	24#	n.a.
Zwergel 1995	214	3.2	n.a.	n.a.	3.9
Horninger 1996	1211	7.6	n.a.	n.a.	5.6
Gallucci 1998	80	3.8	0.0	5.0	3.8
Gilling 1999	59	3.2	6.6	8.2	9.8
Borboroglu 1999	520	n.a.	2.5	2.1	3.1
Kuntz 2004	100	5.0	3.0	10.5	2.2
Muzzonigro 2004	113	1.8	n.a.	n.a.	3.6

Table 22.3 Late complications after TURP- comparison of two decades

n.a. = not available; 22% preoperative impotent

ejaculatory duct) is spared during resection. More importantly, in case of younger patients, the indication for TURP should be taken carefully versus medical treatment with alpha-blockers or 5-alpha-reductase-inhibitors, and even a transurethral incision of the prostate (TUIP). However, preservation of antegrade ejaculation in selected patients is possible.

22.6.9 Erectile dysfunction

The use of HF-generated current close to the capsule may lead to damage of the neurovascular bundles. The rate of impotence varies from 3.4–32 % in the literature.

> However, there are also reports of improved erections following TURP.

The controversy on erectile dysfunction after TURP was clarified by the VA cooperative study group comparing TURP with watchful waiting: After a follow-up of almost 3 years, the proportion of patients reporting deterioration of sexual performance was identical in both arms (19 vs. 21 %), whereas 3 % in each group reported improvement of erectile dysfunction. Today the rate ranges from 2.1 to 11 % in the reviewed literature (Table 22.3). However, it has to be mentioned, that none of these studies used a validated questionnaire (i.e. IEEF-score) for evaluation of impotence.

22.6.10 Recurrent BPH

Re-treatment rate of TURP is lower than those of other primary non-deobstructive treatment alternatives (i.e. TUMT, TUNA) lying in the range of 3–14.5 % after 5 years. Reasons for Re-TURP include insufficient resection as well as the natural course of the disease. This issue might become more important, when laser ablation or vaporization techniques have been performed. Depending on the preferred technique, re-treatment rates of 5–20% can be expected.

22.7 Associated morbidity and mortality

Despite the increasing mean age of the patients (i.e. 55 % > 70 years), the associated morbidity of TURP maintained a similar low range of less than 1% with a mortality rate of 0-0.25% in large series. It has to be mentioned, that nevertheless, TURP has still to be taken seriously, particularly in case of cardiac disease, and that coagulation disorders should be checked preoperatively (i.e. no use of aspirine).

In conclusion, the morbidity of contemporary TURP is lower than previously reported. This is based on a continuously improving armamentarium and technique, but also related to a significant improvement in teaching modalities, including Video-technology (i.e. Video-TUR), hands-on courses with phantoms, TURP-courses with live-demonstrations, and textbooks with CDrom demonstrating the different steps of the technique.

References

Berger AP, Wirtenberger W, Bektic J, Steiner H, Spranger R, Bartsch G, Horninger W (2004) Safer transurethral resection of the prostate: coagulating intermittent cutting reduces hemostatic complications *J Urol* **171**: 289–91.

Borboroglu PG, Kane CJ, Ward JF, Roberts JL, Sands JP (1999) Immediate and postoperative complications of transurethral prostatectomy in the 1990s *J Urol* **162**: 1307–10.

Doll HA, Black NA, McPherson K, Flood AB, Williams GB, Smith JC (1992) Mortality, morbidity and complications following transurethral resection of the prostate for benign prostatic hypertrophy *J Urol* **147**: 1566–73.

Galluci M, Puppo P, Perachino M, Fortunato P, Muto G, Mandressi A, Comeri G, Boccafoschi, Francesca F, Guazzzieri S, Pappagallo GL (1998) Transurethral electrovaporization of the prostate vs transurethral resection *Eur Urol* **33**: 359–64.

Gilling PJ, Mackey M, Cresswell M, Kennett K, Kabalin JN, Fraundorfer MR (1999) Holmium laser versus transurethral resection of the prostate: a randomized prospective trial with 1-year followup *J Urol* **162**: 1640–4.

Hartung R, Leyh H, Liapi C, Fastenmeier K, Barba M (2001) Coagulating intermittent cutting Improved high-frequency surgery in transurethral prostatectomy *Eur Urol* **39**: 676–81.

Haupt G, Pannek J, Benkert S, Heinrich C, Schulze H, Senge (1997) T: Transurethral resection of the prostate with microprocessor controlled electrosurgical unit *J Urol* **158**: 497.

Heidler H (1999) Frequency and causes of fluid absorption: a comparison of three techniques for resection of the prostate under continuous pressure monitoring *BJU Int* **83**: 619–22.

Horninger W, Unterlechner H, Strasser H, Bartsch G (1996) Transurethral prostatectomy: mortality and morbitidy *Prostate* **28**: 195–8.

Kuntz RM, Ahyai S, Lehrich K, Fayad A (2004) Transurethral holmium laser enucleation of the prostate versus transurethral electrocautery resection of the prostate: a randomized prospective trial in 200 patients *J Urol* **172**: 1012–16.

Madersbacher S, Marberger M (1999) Is transurethral resection of the prostate still justified? *BJU Int* **83**: 227–37.

Mebust WK, Holtrgreve HL, Cockett ATK, Peters PC (1989) Transurethral prostatectomy: Immediate and postoperative complications A cooperative study of 13 participating institutions evaluating 3,885 patients *J Urol* **141**: 243–7.

Muzzonigro G, Milanese G, Minardi D, Yehia M, Galosi AB, Dellabella M (2004) Safety and efficacy of transurethral resection of prostae glands up to 150 ml: a prespective comparative study with 1 year of follow up *J Urol* **172**: 611–15.

Rassweiler J, Teber D, Kuntz R, Hofmann R (2006) Complications of transurethral resection of the prostate (TURP)—incidence, management and prevention *Eur. Urol* **50**: 969–80.

Reich O. Gratzke C, Bachmann A, Seitz M, Schlenker B, Hermanek P, Lack N, Stief CG (2008) Morbidity, mortality and early outcome of transurethral resection of the prostate: a prospective multicenter evaluation of 10,654 patients *J Urol* **180**(1): 246–9.

Wasson JH, Reda DJ, Bruskewitz RC, Ellison J, Kelly N, Henderson WG (1995) for the Veterans affairs cooperative study group on transurethral resection of the prostate *N Engl J Med* **322**: 75–9.

Westenberg A, Gilling P, Kennett K, Frampton C, Fraundorfer M (2004) Homium laser resection of the prostate versus transurethral resection of the prostate: results of a randomized trial with 4-year minimum long-term follow up *J Urol* **172**: 616–19.

Zwergel U, Wullich B, Lindenmeir U, Rohde V, Zwergel T (1998) Long-term results following transurethral resection of the prostate *Eur Urol* **33**: 476–80.

Chapter 23

Algorithms in the management of benign prostatic hyperplasia

Judith Dockray and Gordon Muir

Key points

- Benign prostatic hyperplasia (BPH) is the commonest cause of lower urinary tract symptoms (LUTS) in the aging male
- Management is guided by patient's symptoms
- Often a sequential process of escalating treatment that is accelerated if the patient presents with a complication of BPH, e.g. AUR
- Newer minimally invasive treatments are more acceptable to patients than traditional invasive procedures but long-term data on re-operation rates are awaited
- Algorithms in both primary and specialist care allow rapid adoption of EBM with minimal effort, improving standardization of treatment and avoiding unnecessary interventions and cost.

Benign prostatic hyperplasia is a progressive disease, increasing in incidence with age. The incidence and severity of LUTS caused by BPH also increases with age. As the impact of LUTS on quality of life scores (QoL) is subjective, it is often patient choice that determines treatment threshold unless a patient develops a complication of BPH that makes more invasive treatments a necessity.

Due to the multi-factorial aetiology of BPH, it is difficult to predict how patients will progress and who will develop complications.

The Algorithms presented are based on evidence-based assessments of a number of symptoms and risk factors which are briefly summarised before discussion of the algorithms themselves. Symptoms have been discussed elsewhere, (see Chapter 3).

23.1 **Risk factors**

Risk factors for progression are:
- Increasing age
- Raised or rising prostate specific antigen (PSA)
- Larger prostate volume
- Low maximum flow rate (Qmax)
- High post void residual volume (PVR)
- Severity of LUTS (subjective) and dynamic changes in these over time.

23.2 **Treatment options**

23.2.1 **Watchful waiting**

This is suitable for men with low symptom scores on either the International Prostate Symptom Score (IPSS) or American Urological Association Score (AUA Score), and low risk of progression. In young men this strategy should considered first.

23.2.2 **Lifestyle advice**

This is an area with little research, but there is consensus on the following points:

1. Decrease fluid intake, especially at night (to prevent nocturia) and when out of the house, but do not go below 1500ml/day to protect renal function
2. Avoidance or decrease of caffeine and alcohol intake
3. Relaxation and double voiding techniques
4. Distraction techniques—penile squeezing, breathing exercises, perineal pressure
5. Bladder re-training
6. Overhaul of concomitant medication that may affect urinary symptoms
7. Treatment of constipation.

23.2.3 **Phytotherapy**

There is evidence of some symptom benefit with certain plant extracts which are more used in some countries than others.

23.2.4 **Medical treatment**

This is the treatment of choice for moderate to severe LUTS with a low risk of progression to the complications of BPH.

23.2.4.1 *Alpha-1-Adrenoreceptor antagonists (A1-ARAs)*

All alpha blockers improve urine flow and may improve storage symptoms by inhibition of A1-ARs in bladder smooth muscle. Regarding efficacy all available A1-ARAs are comparable, but they differ slightly in side-effects. They have a rapid onset, so will show benefit within one month or should be discontinued.

They are effective on all prostate volumes, and have low long-term side effects. However, they do not halt disease progression or affect risk of retention and symptoms recur on stopping treatment.

23.2.4.2 *Anticholinergic medications*

If storage symptoms are a particular issue, anti-muscarinics can be added as combination therapy if there is no significant residual volume post micturition, due to risk of retention. If erectile dysfunction is a problem a PDE 5 inhibitor can be added but beware of the risk of hypotension with the combination of these two.

23.2.4.3 *5-alpha reductase inhibitors (5ARI)*

These act by inhibiting 5-alpha reductase.So 5ARIs can decrease gland size by 20–30% over 2 years, decrease symptom score by 25% after starting decreasing volume, can be used for haematuria associated with BPH, and can be used for large prostates with or without subsequent surgery.

However, they have a relatively slow onset of actionand may take up to 6 months to see maximal effect. Research into their place in suppression or progression of prostate cancer is ongoing.

23.2.5 **Combination treatment.**

Several studies (MTOPS and CombAT-trial) have shown modest improvements in a combination of alpha blocker plus 5-ARI compared with monotherapy, although cost may be a factor to consider, and the combination of two drugs does not appear to approach the efficacy of surgery.

Therefore combination treatment is usually restricted to patients with LUTS, with larger prostate volume and at risk of progression who wish to avoid surgery.

Indication for medical treatment (e.g. A1-ARA, 5-ARI's) in patients with LUTS due to BPH should always be balanced to the potential risk of increasing perioperative complications with delayed surgery. There is no justification of prolonged medical treatment in patients in whom an initial medical trial failed.

23.2.6 **Surgical treatment**

This is indicated if LUTS are refractory to medical treatment or if the patient declines medical treatment or there is BPH with complications of:

• Acute or chronic urinary retention
• Recurrent urinary retention
• Recurrent haematuria refractory to 5ARI
• Renal insufficiency or
• Bladder stones/large bladder diverticula.

Surgery which creates a prostate cavity will in general give improvements in flow rates of around 100%, voiding rates in retention greater than 95%, and symptom score improvements of 50% or greater. The methods of achieving this are discussed elsewhere in this book, and the patient's severity of symptoms and co-morbidity may guide the algorithm-driven choice of surgical technique.

23.3 **Algorithms for BPH management**

Medical algorithms tend to give a pictorial distillation of evidence based practice reviewed by a panel of experts. A number of algorithms have been proposed for BPH management and tend to be aimed at the primary care physician. However there is no reason to believe that promoting easily digested EBM should not be expanded to specialist care.

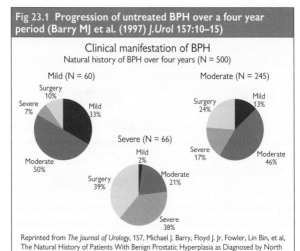

Fig 23.1 Progression of untreated BPH over a four year period (Barry MJ et al. (1997) *J.Urol* **157:10–15)**

Clinical manifestation of BPH
Natural history of BPH over four years (N = 500)

Mild (N = 60)
Surgery 10%
Severe 7%
Mild 33%
Moderate 50%

Moderate (N = 245)
Surgery 24%
Mild 13%
Moderate 46%
Severe 17%

Severe (N = 66)
Mild 2%
Moderate 21%
Surgery 39%
Severe 38%

Reprinted from *The Journal of Urology*, 157, Michael J. Barry, Floyd J. Jr. Fowler, Lin Bin, et al, The Natural History of Patients With Benign Prostatic Hyperplasia as Diagnosed by North American Urologists, Copyright (1997), with permission from Elsevier.

In each of the algorithms listed, regular updates are made available by the organization concerned and are available on the internet links referenced by each diagram.

In understanding the algorithms, initial reference to the guidelines on BPH produced by the relevant bodies will be helpful to the specialist and family physician alike, and at present these are freely available on line.

When patients are questioning the choice of algorithm driven treatment, we often find it useful to let them have an idea of the likely natural history of untreated BPH as described in the longitudinal study reported by Barry and colleagues in 1997 (Figure 23.1). This, as with the available algorithms, relies heavily on the symptom score to predict disease progression and guide management.

With regard to the various different algorithms available, we have chosen to reproduce two based on the EBM guidelines, one for

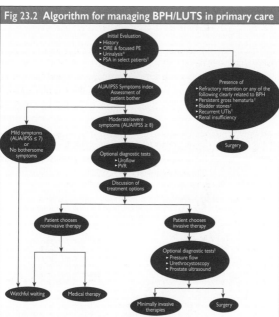

Fig 23.2 Algorithm for managing BPH/LUTS in primary care

Initial Evaluation
▶ History
▶ DRE & focused PE
▶ Urinalysis*
▶ PSA in select patients†

AUA/IPSS Symptoms index
Assessment of
patient bother

Presence of
▶ Refractory retention or any of the
 following clearly related to BPH
▶ Persistent gross hematuria‡
▶ Bladder stones‡
▶ Recurrent UTIs‡
▶ Renal insufficiency

Moderate/severe
symptoms (AUA/IPSS ≥ 8)

Mild symptoms
(AUA/IPSS ≤ 7)
or
No bothersome
symptoms

Surgery

Optional diagnostic tests
▶ Uroflow
▶ PVR

Discussion of
treatment options

Patient chooses
noninvasive therapy

Patient chooses
invasive therapy

Optional diagnostic tests§
▶ Pressure flow
▶ Urethrocystoscopy
▶ Prostate ultrasound

Watchful waiting   Medical therapy

Minimally invasive
therapies

Surgery

*In patients with clinically significant prostatic bleeding, a course of a 5 alpha-reductase inhibitor may be used. If bleeding persists, tissue ablative surgery is indicated.
†Patients with at least a 10-year life expectancy for whom knowledge of the presence of prostate cancer would change management or patients for whom the PSA measurement may change the management of voiding symptoms.
‡After exhausting other therapeutic options as discussed in detail in the text.
§Some diagnostic tests are used in predicting response to therapy. Pressure-flow studies are most useful in men prior to surgery.

AUA, American Urological Association; DRE, digital rectal exam; IPSS, International Prostate Symptom Score; PE, physical exam; PSA, prostate-specific antigen; PVR, postvoid residual urine; UTI, urinary tract infection.

Image reprinted with permission from eMedicine.com, 2010. Available at: http://emedicine.medscape.com/article/445105-overview.

primary care and one for specialists. There are few significant differences between them, any variance being in small detail. Essentially both algorithms will guide a patient with minimal symptoms down a conservative route in the first instance, while for patients with moderate symptoms a trial of medical therapy is the norm. For patients with severe symptoms the choice lies between medical therapy or surgery, with an emphasis on re-evaluation of treatment effect in these patients who do not have a physical therapy. Both algorithms attempt to select those patients with "absolute" indications for surgery early in the decision making process.

Algorithms offer a simple way of managing patients in a logical and evidence based fashion. While particularly useful in primary care assessment and management of lower urinary tract symptoms, urologists will also find them a useful tool for validating their management plans and informing patients.

References

de la Rosette J, Alivizatos G, Madersbacher S, Rioja Sanz C, Nordling J, Emberton M, Gravas S, Michel MC, Oelke M (2006) *European Association of Urology Guidelines on Benign Prostatic Hyperplasia*, European Association of Urology.

Kaplan SA (2006) Update on the American Urological Association Guidelines for the Treatment of Benign Prostatic Hyperplasia *Rev Urol* **8**(4): S10–17.

Lourenco T, Pickard R, Vale L, Grant A, Fraser C, MacLennan G, N'Dow J (2008) Minimally invasive treatments for benign prostatic enlargement: systematic review of randomised control trials *BMJ* **337**: 1662.

Schneider T (2008) Lower urinary tract symptoms suggestive of benign prostatic hyperplasia: prevention or retention? *Eur Urol* **7**: 696–701.

Shahin O (2008) When to treat the prostate, the bladder, or both? *Eur Urol* **7**: 690–5.

Speakman MJ (2008) Lower urinary tract symptoms suggestive of benign prostatic hyperplasia (LUTS/BPH): more than treating symptoms? *Eur Urol* **7**: 680–9.

Van Kerrebroeck P (2008) Back to the future: introduction and conclusions *Eur Urol* **7**: 675–9.

Chapter 24

Emergencies due to BPH

Stephen F. Wyler and Malte Rieken

> ### Key points
> - Acute urinary retention necessitates immediate drainage of the bladder
> - In acute prostatitis antibiotic treatment and depending on severity hospitalization is necessary
> - In case of infection concomitant urological disorders need to be treated immediately
> - Urethral strictures are often related to prior transurethral intervention.

24.1 Prostatitis

Prostatitis is a disease entity affecting 10 to 14% of men. One out of two men will suffer from prostatitis during their life. Bacterial prostatitis is diagnosed clinically and by evidence of inflammation and infection localized in the prostate. Depending on the duration of symptoms, prostatitis can be differentiated into acute and chronic if symptoms persist for more than three months.

Bacterial prostatitis has to be distinguished from chronic pelvic pain syndrome (CPPS), in which no infective agent can be detected and aetiology is multifactorial in most cases. While acute prostatitis is a urologic emergency, chronic prostatitis often is characterized by an undulant clinical course.

24.1.1 Aetiology of acute prostatitis

Bacterial infection of the prostate can be caused by ascending urethral infection, influx of infected urine into prostatic ducts, or by invasion of rectal bacteria after prostate biopsy with lymphogenous or haematogenous spread. Indwelling transurethral catheters are associated with an increased risk of acute prostatitis.

- The most common uropathogen causing acute prostatitis is *Escherichia coli*, which accounts for approximately 75% of all cases

- *Enterobacteriaceae* such as *Klebsiella*, *Enterobacteria*, *Proteus* and *Serratia* are detected frequently
- Mycobacterial, fungal, or viral prostatitis are rare

24.1.2 **Diagnosis and treatment of acute prostatitis**

The diagnosis of acute prostatitis generally does not pose any difficulties. The patient usually complains of an abrupt onset of constitutional symptoms like:

- Fever and chills
- Malaise
- Arthralgia or myalgia
- Rectal or perineal pain.

Moreover, urinary symptoms may be present like:

- Frequency
- Urgency
- Dysuria.

Digital rectal exam reveals a swollen prostate which is painful on palpation. Thus, prostate massage is contraindicated in these cases as it may cause pain and can lead to sepsis. The causing bacteria are mainly gram negative and can be isolated from the urine. Once diagnosed, empiric treatment with antibiotics should be initiated in all cases and can be life-saving.

- Principally, the use of Guidelines of the European Association of Urology (Grabe et al., 2009) is recommended if the parenteral administration of high doses of bactericidal antibiotics is necessary
- Broad-spectrum penicillin, third-generation cephalosporin or fluoroquinolone can be administered and initially can be combined with an aminoglycoside.
- Once the results of bacterial susceptibility testing are available and infection parameters and symptoms have normalized, the administration have to be changed to oral and given for two to four weeks in total.
- In case of postvoid residual urine or acute urinary retention, bladder drainage with a suprapubic catheter is necessary.
- If a prostatic abscess is present, drainage by transurethral resection can be necessary.

24.2 **Urinary retention**

Acute urinary retention (AUR) is a common urological emergency. It is characterized by a sudden and mostly painful inability to void. The annual incidence of primary AUR varies from around two to six per 1000 men and is dependent on age. As up to one third of all men undergoing transurethral resection of the prostate (TURP) are in retention, AUR is an important public health and economic issue.

24.2.1 Aetiology of acute urinary retention

Several aetiological and pathogenic mechanisms have been suggested as possible causes of AUR (Table 24.1):

- An increased resistance to the urinary flow either caused by mechanical or dynamic obstruction
- Bladder over-distension which can be secondary to the influence of drugs like anticholinergics, opiates, or opioides
- Neuropathic causes.
- Trauma.

In most cases, AUR simply is the consequence of the natural course of BPH. Several risk factors have been identified as being associated with an increased risk of AUR and BPH-related surgery. Convincing scientific evidence shows that BPH is a progressive disease in many men and can affect their quality of life. Since surveys have shown that the majority of BPH patients are concerned about AUR and prostate-related surgery, it is important to identify patients at risk.

The most extensively studied factors indicating BPH progression are age, prostate volume (PV) and serum PSA:

- Several studies have demonstrated a correlation between age and BPH progression
- Men with a PV equal to or larger than 30 ml are significantly more likely to suffer moderate to severe symptoms, decreased flow rates, AUR and BPH-related surgery compared with men with a PV smaller than 30 ml
- Since there is a correlation between PV and serum PSA, increased PSA levels are associated with an increased risk of BPH progression
- Recent studies have shown that other variables such as symptom scores and PVR volume are predictors of AUR in men with BPH.

Furthermore, AUR can be triggered by various other conditions or events such as:

- Pain, general or regional anaesthesia, immobility
- Increased alcohol intake
- Urinary tract infection, acute prostatitis.

24.2.2 Management of acute urinary retention

In clinical routine, a suprapubic catheter only is used if transurethral drainage fails. Suprapubic drainage can be associated with a higher risk of haematuria or catheter obstruction, while the rate of urinary tract infection and urethral strictures is significantly lower.

Furthermore, a suprapubic catheter has the advantage that it can be easily closed for a trial without catheter (TWOC) rather than the transurethral catheter being removed and reinserted in case of failure.

Table 24.1	
Cause	Incidence (%)
BPH natural history (spontaneous AUR)	70.3
Postoperative (with general or locoregional anaesthesia	11.2
Important alcohol intake	3.5
Faecal impaction	3.3
Medications (parasympatholytics, sympathomimetics, etc.)	2.8
Need to postpone voiding (travelling by car, immobilization, etc.)	2.4
Acute ano-rectal pain	2.2
Urinary tract infection	2.0
Acute medical condition (cardiac failure, etc.)	0.4
Urolithiasis	0.3
Other	1.6

Based on data from: Emberton M, and Fitzpatrick JM (2008) The Reten-World survey of the management of acute urinary retention: preliminary results *BJU Int*

The initial management of AUR consists of immediate bladder drainage with transurethral or suprapubic catheterization, unless of the reason.

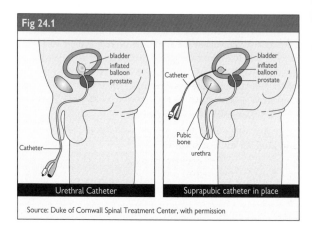

Fig 24.1

Source: Duke of Cornwall Spinal Treatment Center, with permission

After catheterization the patients are either hospitalized or managed in an outpatient setting depending on local practice. After several days of drainage a TWOC is performed:

- Frequently patients receive α_1-blockers like alfuzosin, tamsulosin or doxazosin before catheter removal. The rationale is that AUR might develop due to stimulation of α_1-adrenergic receptors. Bladder outlet resistance can be reduced by decreasing the high sympathetic tone at the level of the urethra and the bladder neck, thus facilitating normal voiding

- Several studies have shown that α_1-blockade before TWOC is associated with a higher success rate

- In case of successful TWOC patients should continue α_1-blockade and be followed regularly

- Whenever the patient is at high risk for BPH progression, the addition of a 5α-reductase inhibitor or surgery should be discussed

- If a TWOC fails, BPH-related surgery or continuous bladder drainage with a suprapubic catheter is necessary.

24.3 Urethral stricture/bladder neck stricture

A urethral stricture is an abnormal narrowing of the urethra which can be symptomatic, asymptomatic, nonobstructive or obstructive. Generally, a urethral narrowing does not get symptomatic unless it is 18 French or less.

Urethral stricture and bladder neck stricture lead to a deterioration of urine flow, increase of voiding symptoms and postvoid residual volume and might be the reason for AUR. In relation to BPH, urethral stricture and bladder neck stricture occur in general as a result of surgery.

> A bladder neck stricture is an abnormal narrowing of the bladder neck, leading to an obstruction of urine flow once progressing.

24.3.1 Aetiology and diagnosis of urethral strictures and bladder neck strictures

In the context of BPH, urethral and bladder neck strictures can occur as a result of transurethral surgery. After TURP, the rate of urethral strictures ranges from around 2–10%. Meatal strictures mostly occur as a consequence of an inappropriate relationship between the diameter of the urethral meatus and the size of the operation instrument, whereas bulbar urethral strictures mostly occur due to insufficient insulation by the lubricant leading to a leakage of the monopolar current.

- To avoid urethral strictures during transurethral surgery, the gel should be applied carefully to the urethra and the shaft of the instrument
- Gel should be reapplied in case of a longer intervention and a high cutting current should be avoided
- An internal urethrotomy should be performed before TURP in case of pre-existing strictures
- Patients with glands smaller than 30 ml tend to develop bladder neck strictures with a higher frequency than patients with larger glands
- The incidence can be reduced by a simultaneous bladder neck incision during TURP.

Diagnosis of urethral and bladder neck strictures includes basic

> Bladder neck strictures occur after TURP with an incidence of up to 9%. One of the major reasons are inappropriate opening if the bladder neck combined with an extensive adenoma resection in small prostates. Additionally a too strong coagulation at the bladder neck has to be avoided.

evaluation like urine flow analysis and abdominal ultrasound including determination of PVR. Furthermore, cystoscopy and in case of a urethral stricture a retrograde urethrography are necessary to determine the localisation and length of the stricture.

24.3.2 **Treatment of urethral strictures and bladder neck strictures**

Short bulbar strictures can be treated with visual internal urethrotomy or dilatation with a cure rate of around 50%. Since open urethroplasty has produced superior results with a long-term recurrence rate of around 15%, there is a clear trend towards primary urethral reconstruction.

> The treatment of urethral strictures depends on the localisation and length of the stricture.

If a patient develops a recurrent stricture after urethrotomy or dilatation, the only curative therapy is an open urethroplasty. Furthermore, in case of longer strictures, an urethroplasty shows the highest success rate. If the stricture is one centimetre or less in length, an anastomotic urethroplasty is usually performed. In longer strictures a substitution urethroplasty with flap or graft is necessary. Bladder neck strictures are usually treated with transurethral electrical or laser incision of the bladder neck. Howerver, recurrent bladder neck strictures occur often.

24.4 Sepsis/urinary tract infection

Patients with urinary tract infection (UTI) may develop sepsis, this being a severe and potentially life-threatening systemic response to infection.

24.4.1 Aetiology of urinary tract infection

Micro-organisms can reach the urinary tract by haematogenous or lymphatic spread, but the most common cause for UTI is the ascent of micro-organisms from the urethra, especially organisms of enteric origin (E. coli and other Enterobacteriaceae).

Candida albicans can cause UTI via the haematogenous route or as ascending infection after antibiotic therapy.

24.4.2 Diagnosis and treatment of urinary tract infection

The diagnosis of urinary tract infection is established by clinical symptoms, results of selected laboratory tests and evidence of the presence of microbes by culturing or other specific tests.

- The number of bacteria is considered relevant for diagnosis of a UTI, in men $\geq 10^4$ colony-forming units of uropathogen/ml of mid-stream sample of urine is relevant
- In a suprapubic bladder puncture specimen, any count of bacteria is relevant
- In patients with complicating factors for UTI a positive urine culture and an underlying urological disorder can be found:
  - Presence of an indwelling catheter or stent
  - Post-void residual urine >100 ml
  - Obstructive uropathy of any aetiology like stones or tumours
  - Perioperative and postoperative UTI.

In UTI with complicating factors the spectrum of bacteria is larger and they are more likely to be resistant to antimicrobial therapy. Whereas the treatment of ordinary UTI necessitates 3–10 days of antibiotic therapy, in UTI with complicating factors the underlying urological disorder needs to be managed simultaneously with antibiotic treatment.

If empirical antibiotic therapy has to be performed, mostly fluoroquinolones, aminopenicillin with -lactam inhibitor, a group 2 or 3a cephalosporin or in the case of parenteral therapy, an aminoglycoside are recommended for 7–14 (-21) days.

24.4.3 Aetiology, diagnosis and treatment of sepsis

Sepsis is diagnosed when clinical evidence of UTI is accompanied by signs of systemic inflammation. The systemic inflammatory response syndrome (SIRS: fever or hypothermia, hyperleucocytosis or leucopenia, tachycardia, tachypnoea) is recognized as the first event in a cascade to multi-organ failure, therefore early diagnosis and inter-disciplinary treatment is crucial.

Treatment of urosepsis:

- Immediate drainage of any obstruction in the urinary system or management of underlying urologic disorder
- If an internal drainage of the bladder or kidney via transure-thral catheter or ureteric stent is not possible a percutaneous drainage with suprapubic catheter or percutaneous nephrostomy has to be performed
- Life-supporting care, antibiotic therapy and adjunctive measures (sympathomimetic amines, hydrocortisone, blood glucose control, recombinant activated protein C).

References

Emberton M, Cornel EB, Bassi PF, Fourcade RO, Gómez JM, Castro R (2008) Benign prostatic hyperplasia as a progressive disease: a guide to the risk factors and options for medical management *Int J Clin Pract.* **62**(7): 1076–86.

Fitzpatrick JM, Kirby RS (2006) Management of acute urinary retention *BJU Int* **97**(2): 16–20.

Grabe M, Bishop MC, Bjerklund-Johansen TE, Botto H, Cek M, Naber KG, Palou J, Tenke P, Wagenlehner F (2009) *Guidelines on Urological Infections*, European Association of Urology.

Meeks JJ, Erickson BA, Granieri MA, Gonzalez CM (2009) Stricture recur-rence after urethroplasty: a systematic review *J Urol* **182**(4): 1266–70.

Naber KG (2008) Management of bacterial prostatitis: what's new? *BJU Int* **101**(3): 7–10.

Index

A

α_1-adrenoceptor
  receptor agonists
    (ARBs) 90–1, 165
  formulations and
    standard doses 87t
  side effects 87–8
  symptom
    reduction 86–7
α-blockers (ABs) 34,
  86–93, 140, 142
5α-reductase
  inhibitors (ARIs) 88–9,
    165
  formulations and
    standard doses 89
  side effects 89
AAH see atypical
  adenomatous
  hyperplasia (AAH)
Abrams-Griffiths
  nomogram 44, 45f
ABs see α-blockers (ABs)
acute urinary
  retention (AUR)
    aetiology of 171, 172t
    BPH, progression of 3,
      13, 55–6
    management of 171
    TWOC, and
      catheterization 171–3
aging men, and LUTS
  BPH, age-
    related 50, 163
  detrusor function,
    impaired 50
  ED 50
  immobility 50
  nocturia 50
  OAB 50
  prevalence with
    age 10–11, 49,
      85, 137–8
  QoL 49
  testosterone levels 50
alcohol
  consumption 54, 81
alfuzosin 34, 56, 57
ALTESS (Alfuzosin 10mg
  once daily Long-Term
  Efficacy And Safety
  Study) 56

American Urological
  Association Symptom
  Index (AUASI) 19–20
ANS see autonomic
  nervous system (ANS)
ARBs see α_1-adrenoceptor
  receptor agonists
  (ARBs)
ARIs see 5α-reductase
  inhibitors (ARIs)
assessment, of BPH see
  diagnosis and
  assessment,
  of BPH
atypical adenomatous
  hyperplasia (AAH) 25
AUA 7 score 44, 61
AUA (American
  Urological Association)
  Guidelines 102
AUASI see American
  Urological Association
  Symptom Index (AUASI)
AUR see acute urinary
  retention (AUR)
autonomic nervous system
  (ANS) 51

B

benign prostatic
  enlargement (BPE)
    and BOO 43
    BPH, differential
      diagnosis of 66, 66t
    BPO, BPE, LUTS
      coherences 4, 7–8
    definition of 2, 38, 43
    prevalence with
      age 137–8
benign prostatic
  hyperplasia (BPH)
    and BOO 4
    BPO, BPE, LUTS
      coherences 4, 7–8
    characteristics of 65
    definition of 2, 38, 43
    differential diagnosis
      of 7–8, 66, 66t
    epidemiology
      of 2–3, 8–9
    pathophysiology of 10
    progression of 3–4

benign prostatic
  obstruction (BPO) 2
    BPH, differential
      diagnosis of 66, 66t
    BPO, BPE, LUTS
      coherences 4, 7–8
    definition of 38, 43
    prevalence with
      age 137–8
    urodynamic
      studies 45–6
    and voiding LUTS 12
biological plausibility,
  theories supporting
    autonomic hyperactivity
      and metabolic
      syndrome
      hypothesis 55
    nitric oxide synthase
      (NOS) theory 55
    pelvic
      atherosclerosis 55
    Rho-kinase activa-
      tion/endothelin
      pathway 55
bipolar plasma vaporization
  of the prostate 105–6
bladder
  and LUTS 12, 13t, 18
  role of 3, 40, 49, 89, 109
bladder cancer 52
bladder neck
  hypertrophy 52
bladder neck stricture 52,
  171–3
bladder outflow
  obstruction (BOO) 2
    Abrams-Griffiths
      nomogram 44, 45f
    assessment of 44–5
    definition of 38, 43
    detrusor overactivity
      (DO) 46
    neurological disorders,
      men with 47
    peak flow rate 44
    postvoidal residual urine
      (PVR) 44
    urodynamic diagnosis
      of 43–4
    urodynamic studies, and
      BPO 45–6
    uroflowmetry 44

BOO see bladder outflow obstruction (BOO)
Botulinum toxin A injection 141
Boyarski Symptom Assessment, LUTS 18
BPE see benign prostatic enlargement (BPE)
BPH see benign prostatic hyperplasia (BPH)
BPO see benign prostatic obstruction (BPO)

C

cardiovascular disease 49
cataract surgery 88
catheterization 171–3
cerebrovascular accidents 51
chronic pelvic pain syndrome (CPPS) 169
CLAP see contact laser ablation of the prostate (CLAP)
CombAT-trial 143, 165
contact laser ablation of the prostate (CLAP) 111
CPPS see chronic pelvic pain syndrome (CPPS)

D

Danish Prostatic Symptom Score (DAN-PSS) 62
detrusor overactivity (DO) 18, 21, 37, 38, 40, 41f, 46, 51
diabetes mellitus type II (DM) 51
diabetic cystopathy 51
diagnosis and assessment, of BPH
 objective parameters
  blood analysis 70–2
  BPH, characteristics of 65
  differential diagnosis 66, 66t
  digito-rectal examination (DRE) 67
  endoscopic evaluation 76
  imaging 75
  questionnaires 68
  urine analysis 69–70
  urodynamic evaluation 76
  uroflowmetry 72–3
  voiding chart 69
 subjective parameters
  quality of life (QoL) assessment 63–64
  questionnaires, selection of 61–2

symptom score, and outcome severity 62–3
symptoms 59–60
digito-rectal examination (DRE) 25, 67
diode laser vaporization of the prostate
 diode laser
  prostatectomy complications 134
  durability 134
  haemostatic properties 133
  interoperative safety 133, 134, 135
 diode lasers, tissue ablation capacities
  coagulation depth 132–3
  penetration depth 132–3, 134
  wavelengths, varying 131
DO see detrusor overactivity (DO)
doxazosin 57, 87, 88
DRE see digito-rectal examination (DRE)
dysuria 22

E

ED see erectile dysfunction (ED)
emergencies, due to BPH
 AUR 170–3
 prostatitis 169–70
 urethral stricture/bladder neck stricture 171–3
 UTIs, and sepsis 175–6
endocrine disease 49
endoscopy 76
epidemiology, of BPH
 histological BPH, prevalence of 8–9
 LUTS 9
erectile dysfunction (ED)
 ABs 34
 age-related changes 33, 50
 ARB, side effects of 88
 ARIs 34
 BPH/LUTS, evidence for association with 33–4
 ejaculatory disorders 34
 nitric oxide/cGMP signalling pathway, role of 33–4
 PDE-5s 33, 34–5, 88
 prevalence of 33
 sildenafil 35
 and TURP 159–60
 vardenafil 35
estrogen receptors (ER) 27

G

gallium-aluminium-arsenide diode lasers 111
greenlight vaporization see KTP-Greenlight laser vaporization

H

Holmium laser treatment, of BHP
 Holmium laser, properties of 122
 Holmium laser ablation of the Prostate (HoLAP) 125
 Holmium laser enucleation of prostate (HoLEP) 112, 121, 141
  haemostatic and incisional properties 122
  learning curve 124–5
  versus prostatectomy 124
  versus TURP 121, 123–4
 HoLRP (Holmium:YAG) laser 112

I

ICIQ-MLUTS assessment, storage symptoms 21–2
ILC see interstitial laser coagulation (ILC)
imaging
 bladder ultrasound 75–6
 prostate ultrasound 76
 renal ultrasound 75
immobility, age-related 50
incontinence, and TURP 157–8
International Continence Society (ICS) 46, 62
International Prostate Symptom Score (IPSS) 21, 44, 102
 BPH, diagnosis and assessment of 4, 68
 reliability of 62–3
interstitial laser coagulation (ILC) 111
IPSS see International Prostate Symptom Score (IPSS)

K

kallikrein see prostatic specific antigen (PSA)
KTP-Greenlight laser vaporization 112
 background 115–16

laser beam tissue
   interactions, types
   of 116
laser penetration
   depth 116
PVP, clinical outcomes
   of 118–20
tissue ablation
   capacities 132–3

L

laser systems see diode
   laser vaporization of
   the prostate; Holmium
   laser treatment, of
   BHP; KTP-Greenlight
   laser vaporization;
   neodymium yttrium-
   aluminium-garnet
   (Nd:YAG) laser
linear passive urethral
   resistance relation
   (LinPURR) 44
lithium triborat (LBO) 112
lower urinary tract
   symptoms (LUTS)
   bladder function 12,
      13t, 18
   and BOO 40
   BPH, differential
      diagnosis of 66, 66t
   definition of 1
   diagnosis of 49
   epidemiology of
      epi-LUTS
         study 11–12
      population-based
         survey 11
      prevalence as
         age-related 11
      urgency 12
   pathophysiologic
      conditions evoking
      bladder cancer 52
      bladder neck
         hypertrophy 52
      cerebrovascular
         accidents 51
      congestive heart
         failure 52
      dementia 51
      diabetes mellitus type
         II (DM) 51
      Parkinson's disease
         (PD) 51
      prostate cancer 52
      transient problems 51
      urethral stricture 52
      urinary tract
         infections 52
   pathophysiology of 12
   postmicturition
      symptoms 2, 11
   prostate cancer,
      fear of 79

prostate
   enlargement 17
   as prostatism 18, 49
   storage LUTS 12, 13t
   types of 12
   voiding LUTS 2, 12
   in women 89
   see also overactive
      bladder (OAB)
LUTS see lower urinary
   tract symptoms (LUTS)

M

Madsen and Iversen BPH
   symptom score 18
management, of BPH
   algorithms for
      BPH, progression of
         untreated over four
         year period 166f
      BPH/LUTS, algorithm
         for management
         of in primary
         care 167f
      BPH/LUTS, algorithm
         for specialist care
         management of 168f
   risk-adapted
      patients at risk 141–4
      senior adults,
         treatment of 138–41
Maximum Flow Rate
   (Qmax) 102, 139
Medical Therapy of
   Prostatic Symptoms
   (MTOPS) 4, 55, 56, 57,
   143, 165
medical treatments
   anticholinergics 89–90,
      140, 165
   ARBs 86–8, 90–1, 165
   ARIs 88–9, 140, 143, 165
   combination
      therapy 91–2, 143
   critical use of 144
   PDE5-inhibitors 90–1
   phytotherapy 85–6,
      140, 142
metabolic syndrome 28–9
modular autonomous
   hypothesis, for OAB 40
MTOPS see Medical
   Therapy of Prostatic
   Symptoms (MTOPS)
multiple system atrophy
   (MSA) 51
muscarinic receptor
   agonists 37, 89–90, 91
myogenic hypothesis,
   for OAB 39

N

natural history, of BPH 4, 7–9
necrosis 134

neodymium yttrium-
   aluminium-garnet
   (Nd:YAG) laser
   CLAP 111
   ILC 111
   laser penetration
      depth 116
   limitations of 115
   TULIP 110
   VLAP 110–111
neurogenic hypothesis, for
   OAB 39
neurological disease 47, 49
nitric oxide synthase
   (NOS) theory 55
nocturia 11, 38, 50, 51
nocturnal polyuria 18, 69
nomograms 44, 45f

O

OAB see overactive bladder
   (OAB)
Olmsted County
   Study 3–4, 9, 56, 138
open prostatectomy
   (OP) 101
overactive bladder (OAB)
   age-related 50
   conservative
      management of 40
   definition of 38
   detrusor overactivity
      (DO) 37, 38, 40, 41f
   epidemiology of
      EPIC population-based
         survey 39
      men versus
         women 37, 39–40
      and LUTS 37, 38, 40
      nocturia 38
   pathophysiology of
      modular autonomous
         hypothesis 40
      myogenic
         hypothesis 39
      neurogenic
         hypothesis 39
      urotheliogenic
         hypothesis 39
   storage
      symptoms 38, 39
   terminology 37–8
   treatment plan 41
   urgency 37, 38, 39
   urodynamical testing 40
   voiding symptoms 38

P

Parkinson's disease (PD) 51
pathophysiology, of BPH
   age dependant,
      BPH as 17
   androgen receptor,
      mutations of 10t

pathophysiology, of BPH
(cont.)
androgens, role of 18
bladder, overactive 17
detrusor
dysfunction 18, 21
dysuria 22
epithelial and stromal
tissue, interactions 10,
17, 26
gross hematuria 22
histological,
BPH as 7, 17, 53
lymphocytic
inflammation 18
Madsen and Iversen
BPH symptom
score 18
nocturnal
polyuria 18, 69
prostate and bladder
interactions 22
prostate
enlargement 17
PCA see prostate cancer
(PCA), risk of
PDE-5 see phosphodi-
esterase-5-inhibitors
(PDE-5)
peak flow rate 44
phosphodiesterase-5-
inhibitors (PDE-5) 33,
34–5, 88, 90–1
photoselective vaporization
of prostate (PVP)
bleeding complications,
reduction in 118
follow-up studies 119
postoperative storage
symptoms 118–19
prostate before/during/
after photoselec-
tive vaporization of
prostate 117, 117f
versus TURP 118–19
see also KTP-Greenlight
laser vaporization
phytotherapy 85–6, 140,
142
PIA see proliferative inflammatory atrophy (PIA)
postmicturition
symptoms 2,
postvoidal residual urine
(PVR) 44
potassium-titanyl-phosphate
see KTP-Greenlight
laser vaporization
progression, of BPH
AUR 3, 13, 142
IPPS 3–4
patients at risk,
defining 141–2
progression of
untreated over four
year period 166f

risk factors for 164
surgery, risk factors
for having 55–6
proliferative inflammatory
atrophy (PIA) 28–9
prostate cancer
(PCA), risk of
androgen
dependency 25
androgen deprivation
therapy 25
atypical adenomatous
hyperplasia
(AAH) 25, 27
chronic
inflammation 28–9
epithelial and stromal
tissue, non malignant
growth of 26
estrogen receptors
(ER) 27
metabolic
syndrome 28–9
proliferative
inflammatory atrophy
(PIA) 28–9
prostate cancer,
risk of 72t
prostatic atrophy 28
prostatic specific antigen
(PSA) 29–30
testosterone
levels 27, 28f
transition zone (TZ),
nodular enlargement
in 25, 27
prostatectomy 55–6
prostatic atrophy 28
prostatic specific antigen
(PSA) 29–30
prostatic volume (PV),
assessment of 9
prostatism, LUTS
as 18, 49
prostatitis, acute
acute versus
chronic 169
aetiology of 169–70
bacterial prostatitis
versus CPPS 169
diagnosis and treatment
of 170
PSA see prostatic specific
antigen (PSA)
PV see prostatic volume
(PV), assessment of
PVP see photoselective
vaporization of
prostate (PVP)

Q

quality of life (QoL), and
LUTS 19, 49, 63–4,
102, 163

R

renal insufficiency 3
risk factors, associated
with BPH
age 54
alcohol consumption 54
alfuzosin 57
androgens 54
biological plausibility,
theories supporting 55
diet 54
doxazosin 57
genetics 54
metabolic syndrome 54
physical activity 55
sexual dysfunction 55
smoking 55
surgery, risk factors for
having 55–7

S

senior adults, treatment of
Botulinum toxin A
injection 141
comorbidity/life
expectancy 138–9
HoLEP 141
laser prostatectomy 141
medical therapy 140
photoselective
vaporization of
prostate (PVP) 141
treatment options 139
TUMT 141
TUNA 141
TURP,
monopolar 140–1
urodynamic
considerations 139
sepsis, and UTIs 175–6
serum-creatinine 72
sildenafil 35
silodosin 87, 88
SIRS (systematic
inflammatory response
syndrome) 175–6
smoking 55
storage symptoms 12
strokes 51
surgery, risk factors for
having 55–7
alfuzosin 56
MTOPS, and
identification of
risk factors 56
Olmsted County Study,
and identification of
risk factors 56
progression, of
BPH 55–6
AUR, and
prostatectomy 55–6
progression
events 55–6

progression
rates 55–6
PSA values 56
surgical therapy
urodynamic studies 45
symptom scores,
and outcome
severity 62–3
age and cultural
factors 62
DAN-PSS (Danish
Prostatic Symptom
Score) 62
International
Continence Society
male questionnaire 62
IPSS, reliability of 62–3
linguistic validation 63
patient reports,
reliability of 62
symptoms, of BPH 61–3
BPH, as
asymptomatic 60
diabetes mellitus 60
heart insufficiency 60
late symptoms/
secondary diseases 60
LUTS 59
medical history,
taking 59
neurological
disorders 60
prostate
enlargement 59
storage symptoms 60
symptom score,
use of 61–2
voiding symptoms 60

T

tamsulosin 34, 87, 88
terazosin 87, 88
testosterone levels 27,
28f, 50
Thulium:YAG laser
(Tm:YAG) 112
advantages and
disadvantages 129
functional results 127–8
incisions, precision
of 127
technique, for laser
prostatectomy 127–8
tolterodine 90
transurethral incision
of the prostate
(TUIP) 104
transurethral resection of
the prostate (TURP)
bipolar 104–5
versus HoLEP 121,
123–4
indications and
contraindications
for 148–9

intraoperative
complications of
balloon-
compression 153
bleeding 109, 118,
151–3
comparison of two
decades 149
extravasation 155
incidence and
type 147–8
late after, two
decades 159t
morbidity and
mortality 160
orifices, injury
of 155–6
micturition
parameters,
improvements in 102
monopolar 140
morbidity and
mortality 103
versus photoselective
vaporization of pros-
tate (PVP) 118–19
postoperative
complications of
bladder neck
stenosis 158
bladder
tamponade 156
BPH, recurrent 160
erectile
dysfunction 159–60
incontinence 157–8
infection 157
management 156
retrograde
ejaculation 158–9
urethral stricture 158
urinary retention 157
re-coagulation 154
resection
techniques 149–50
technical aspects 151
prostatic vessels,
vascular control
of 151
transfusion rates,
decreased 151
TUR, improved
training of 151
technological
modifications 103–4
technology 150
bipolar devices 150
coagulating intermit-
tent cutting 150
electrosection 150
TUR-syndrome 154–5
versus watchful
waiting 80
Transurethral (TUR)
Syndrome 122, 140
diagnosis 154

management 154–5
prevention 155
transurethral ultra-
sound-guided laser
prostatectomy (TULIP)
probe 110
treatment options, for BPH
combination
treatment 165
lifestyle advice 164
medical treatment 165
phytotherapy 164
surgical treatment 166
treatment
thresholds 163
watchful waiting 164
trial without catheter
(TWOC) 171–3
TUIP see transurethral
incision of the prostate
(TUIP)
TULIP see transurethral
ultrasound-guided
laser prostatectomy
(TULIP) probe
TUMT 141
TUNA 141
TUR see Transurethral
(TUR) Syndrome
TURP see transurethral
resection of the
prostate (TURP)
TWOC see trial without
catheter (TWOC)

U

ultrasound 75–6
urethral resistance factor
(URA) 44
urethral stricture 52
aetiology of 173–4
description of 173
diagnosis of 174
treatment of 174
urgency 51
urinary retention see
acute urinary
retention (AUR)
urinary tract infections
(UTIs)
aetiology of 175
diagnosis and
treatment of 175
sepsis, diagnosis
of 175–6
urine analysis
erythrocytes/
haemoglobin 70
glucose 70
leukocytes 69
nitrite 69
urodynamic detrusor
overactivity (DO)
see detrusor
overactivity (DO)

uroflowmetry 44, 72–3
urotheliogenic hypothesis,
    for OAB 39
UTIs see urinary tract
    infections (UTIs)

V

VapoEnucleation 128
VapoResection 128
vardenafil 35

Veterans Affairs study 138
visually assisted laser
    prostatectomy
    (VLAP) 110–111
voiding diaries 61, 69
voiding symptoms 2, 12

W

watchful waiting
    conditions for 79–80

patient selection for 80
self-management 81–3
    outcomes, self-
    management *versus*
    standard care 83
    patient assessment
    prior to 81–2
versus TURP 80